[英]尼古拉斯·詹姆斯 著　朱邦芊 译

牛津通识读本·

癌症

Cancer

A Very Short Introduction

译林出版社

图书在版编目（CIP）数据

癌症/（英）尼古拉斯·詹姆斯（Nicholas James）著；
朱邦芊译. —南京：译林出版社，2020.10（2022.7重印）
（牛津通识读本）
书名原文：Cancer: A Very Short Introduction
ISBN 978-7-5447-8194-7

Ⅰ.①癌… Ⅱ.①尼… ②朱… Ⅲ.①癌－诊疗
Ⅳ.①R73

中国版本图书馆 CIP 数据核字（2020）第 055114 号

著作权合同登记号　图字：10-2013-499 号

癌症　［英国］尼古拉斯·詹姆斯／著　朱邦芊／译

责任编辑　许　丹
装帧设计　景秋萍
校　　对　孙玉兰
责任印制　董　虎

原文出版　Oxford University Press, 2011
出版发行　译林出版社
地　　址　南京市湖南路 1 号 A 楼
邮　　箱　yilin@yilin.com
网　　址　www.yilin.com
市场热线　025-86633278
排　　版　南京展望文化发展有限公司
印　　刷　江苏苏中印刷有限公司
开　　本　890 毫米 ×1260 毫米　1/32
印　　张　8.875
插　　页　4
版　　次　2020 年 10 月第 1 版
印　　次　2022 年 7 月第 3 次印刷
书　　号　ISBN 978-7-5447-8194-7
定　　价　39.00 元

序 言

季加孚

　　能够遇到这样一本书，是非常令人愉悦的。本书篇幅并不长，和《众病之王》这类癌症科普的长篇巨著不是同一个类型，却非常适合当下的阅读习惯。即便利用碎片时间阅读，各章节一口气读完并不辛苦。正如这套丛书的定位，作为肿瘤的"通识"读本，它非常合适。

　　首先其内容确实非常广泛，涵盖了不同瘤种，更是囊括了肿瘤这一话题的各方各面，把这个话题一以贯"通"。大多数人接受的有关肿瘤的信息来自网络等媒体，是在家人或者自己罹患之后才开始从网络上搜索而来的针对某一瘤种，甚至针对某几个新疗法的只言片语。姑且不论是否真实可信，这些信息往往存在片面性。即便作为肿瘤专门从业者，我们也非常担心因为专业细分而导致视野逐步狭隘。这是因为作为肿瘤临床医生，我们总是面对一个个的患者，大多数情况下我们擅长的还只是一到两种肿瘤，于是总难免忘了从不同的视角横向或者纵向去看待我们所面临的肿瘤这一难题，而是尝试用解决一种肿瘤的思路去解决其他肿瘤，用治疗一个患者的心态去看待整个人群。这本书在这方面确实是个非常好的提醒，它涵盖了肿瘤的流行病学、病因、病理、治疗等多方面的内容，甚至还涉及了肿瘤研究、卫生经济学乃至替代疗法等。这些对于提升我们的视角，是不无裨益的。

在现代社会想要获取信息不难，甚至应该说过分容易，但从中筛选可靠的信息并不简单。作为医生，我们能够体会到一个肿瘤患者和其家属在治疗期间可能会遇到多少"坑"，网上充斥着大量谣言，身边道听途说不少偏方或是新疗法，一旦踩进去，恐怕就深陷泥淖很难自拔。这本书作为肿瘤科普读物，做到了科学为基，普及为本，对于广大读者而言显得尤为珍贵。尽管短小精悍，但它的能量和知识密度却很高，能在很短的时间内，让我们对这个话题的知识储备进行扩容，帮助我们从过分的悲观中解脱，建立乐观积极的心态，寻找真正科学、有效的治疗方式。

阅读这本书之前，我心里曾有隐隐担忧，怕它和很多癌症科普书籍一样，是"过去"的书，讲有关癌症研究的大量历史，却对眼前的病人和家属没有太多有用信息。这主要是因为癌症领域的发展与突破在近些年实在是太多了。很多书，特别是翻译的书，由于准备周期长，很难获取最新的肿瘤领域进展。而这本书非常难能可贵的一点在于，它涵盖了非常多的肿瘤领域的"现在的"最新研究进展及成果。例如，我们北京大学肿瘤医院胃肠中心是全国最早开始肿瘤多学科诊疗（MDT）的团队，经过多年努力，逐步形成了规范、系统的MDT传统，获得了非常好的治疗效果，并在国内进行推广。实际上我们能够看到目前国内有不少中心还在摸索，因此，当我看到本书介绍这一最新治疗理念时，既意外又欣慰,同时为本书的读者朋友感到高兴。

对于大多数老百姓而言,接触到新技术相关的网络信息时的态度往往分为两类:要么过度乐观,要么过分悲观。乐观者认为某个新技术能解决肿瘤的大问题,因而很多哪怕不适合使用的患者,也常常会在诊疗过程中向我们打听,因为他们受网络信息影响,抱有过多的期待;悲观者觉得新技术不过昙花一现或是换汤不换药。而本书对于新技术、新方法的介绍在我看来是非常实事求是的。例如机器人手术、免疫治疗、靶向治疗,这些技术手段的来龙去脉都在书中有详实的梳理,从肿瘤医生的角度来看,这些有理有据的介绍描述对于患者而言是最有益的。

说到译林出版社的"牛津通识读本"系列,这本书和丛书里的其他书一样,如果只是阅读中文部分,实在可惜。当然,丛书系列里英文的风格各不相同,本书对于大多数烦恼于英文写作的医生或研究人员来说,是非常好的学习参考资料。作为一名忠实读者,也非常感谢出版社能够组织出版这一系列丛书,让那么多非常好的话题、内容以别样的形式与中国读者见面。

目 录

致 谢

写一本书，哪怕这样一册短小的读本，也是个艰巨的任务。我要感谢妻子艾莉森和家人的帮助和支持，他们给了我写书所需要的时间和空间。还要感谢父母为支持我受教育所做的巨大投入，那往往意味着他们个人要做出极大的牺牲。

癌症问题的规模

癌症很常见，极其常见。2008年，大约有1 270万人确诊罹患癌症，其中790万人死亡，约占所有死亡人数的13%。尽管有人认为，癌症是富裕国家的一种老年病，但这类死亡大约70%都发生在低收入或中等收入国家。罹患癌症的人不分性别、种族和贫富。诊断结果令闻者色变，盖因患上癌症的人不啻是接到了死刑判决（通常的确如此）。这种疾病本身及其治疗均会带来极大的痛苦与忧虑。治疗癌症是全世界医疗卫生系统的一大负担，因为导致过早死亡，癌症也是劳动人口丧失生产力的主要原因。本章将概述癌症问题，重点讨论某些更常见的癌症，以说明全球各地的数字有何差异。能够侵袭如此众多人口的疾病必然会有重大的经济影响，因此，本章还会关注经济和医疗卫生事业之间的一些相互作用的方式，这将是后续章节中进一步研究的主题。对于癌症发病率模式的研究为癌症的病因提供了非常有趣的线索（第二章对此有更全面的阐述）。本章也会谈及某 1
些最惊人的关联。

癌症治疗和癌症研究也是产业活动的重要组成部分。临床试验中的半数药物是用于癌症的；2006年，所有癌症药物的全球市场价值为346亿美元，2008年，这一数字估计达到了480亿。分析师预测，2010年到2015年的增长率将达到每年10%以上。制药业每年花费在研究和开发癌症药物上的支出为65亿到80亿美元。这笔开销让政府和研究慈善机构在癌症药物研发上的投入相形见绌，这可能意味着新药都集中在商业影响最大的领域，而非公共卫生的范畴。拥有成功癌症药物的制药公司均位列全球最庞大的企业之中。生物科技公司就算没有可供上市的产品，但只要拥有一种"尚在研发"的有前途的癌症药物，便可因为该药物有可能在未来的某一天获批上市而身价数十亿美元。2009年，至少有19种抗癌药的销售额超过了10亿美元，就算在最富裕的国家，为患者采购这些药物也令医疗卫生系统不堪重负。

　　另一方面，约有三分之一的癌症患者能够接受的有效治疗极其有限，在最贫穷的国家，这一数字上升到一半以上。展望未来，人口日益老龄化，药价呈上升趋势，我们或许会面临这样的局面：只有最发达国家的最富裕阶层才会得到"最先进"的药物治疗。又或者，对治疗反应的预测更准确，会有助于实现针对个体的治疗选择，从而降低不必要或无效的治疗成本。打个比方，我们每次使用汽车或电脑，都预判它们可以运转，癌症药物则不同，大多数药物只对一部分患者有效。对那些以缓解症状或改善生活质量为目标的晚期患者而言，该比例或许远低于50%，因此大多数治疗都是无谓的，实际上或许比无效更糟，因为那些治疗还可能会导致无益的副作用。能够在治疗之前确认哪些患者会从中获益，将会非常节约成本，临床方面也会收效甚佳，因而已成为当今癌症研究的一大重点（见第四和第五章）。

癌症也令全世界的学术机构和大学为之着迷。1961年，约翰·F. 肯尼迪承诺在那个十年结束之前把人送上月球。九年后，尼尔·阿姆斯特朗和巴兹·奥尔德林便漫步于月球之上。十年后的1971年，理查德·尼克松为呼应这一承诺，宣布对癌症"开战"。就像近来的"反恐战争"一样，与一个多面向的全球问题为敌，充其量也不过只获得了局部胜利。尼克松最初承诺花费约一亿美元，这在当时看来简直是天文数字，但结果只是杯水车薪。自1971年以来，后续又投入了数十亿美元的研究经费，但三十多年后，癌症仍是全球最大的致死原因之一，发达国家约三分之一的患者，西方约五分之一的患者死于此病。治疗癌症显然比尖端的"火箭科学"更难。

全球各地为研究癌症的病因和治疗投入了巨额资金。2009—2010年，美国国家癌症研究所花费了47亿美元用于癌症研究；欧洲的相应开销约为14亿欧元。在英国，开支最大的是英国癌症研究中心，该中心是英国最大的慈善机构之一，2010年的捐赠收入超过了5亿英镑，反映出普通大众对找到癌症起因和治疗方案的重视程度（然而公共捐款的最大受助者竟然是动物而非人类！）。虽然研究开支如此庞大，我们还是没有真正理解绝大部分癌症的病因。此外，尽管药物和药物研究所费不赀，事实上却如第三章所述，大多数被治愈的癌症患者要么是因为接受了外科手术，要么是采取了放射疗法。化学疗法和诸如单克隆抗体或靶向"小分子"疗法等新式疗法虽然日益受到重视，其治愈病患的案例仍属少数，但在缓解疾病晚期症状方面却起到

3

3 了重要的作用。

　　看待癌症带来的问题有不同的角度,从原始数据——有多少人确诊,多少人死亡——到个体差异——患上某种具体癌症的个人风险如何?基于人口的统计数据可能会以不同的方式呈现,从整个人口的患病率,到按年龄调整的患病率,再到寿命损失年数的计算。最后这种统计数据通常表示为70岁(《圣经》所说的"三个二十年又加十年")之前的损失年数,因而假设70岁(有时是75岁)之后的死亡基本上代表了因衰老而过世。更复杂的是,癌症死亡率因收入、种族和居住国而大不相同。例如在欧洲和北美,乳腺癌和前列腺癌比日本和中国常见得多。从这些国家去美国的移民患上这些癌症的风险会接近美国白人的发病率,但整体风险仍会保持在较低的水平。这表明,远东地区乳腺癌和前列腺癌的较低发病率,部分原因在于环境,部分原因在于种族差异,或是环境的某些可转移的相关方面,比如日常饮食。

　　为了进一步探讨这些概念,我会使用一系列方法来描述原始统计数据的样本。至于哪些统计数据最有用,取决于读者的视角。例如,在公共卫生领域工作、负责为本地人口规划医疗保健的医生,就不会对另一个国家某种特定癌症的发病率有多少兴趣。相反,着眼于饮食对患癌风险之影响的研究者也许很希望关注不同群体之间发病率的差异,因为它们或许能解释哪些生活方式因素对于某种特定癌症的发展影响较大。癌症研究的资金筹集者倾向于关心目标捐赠人口中患者众多的疾病——在欧洲和北美,这方面的最佳范例就是乳腺癌,但近年来,为前列腺癌筹资的活动也以同样的方式利用了舆论风向。

4

原始数字

如前所述,全世界归因于癌症的死亡占比是13%左右,也就是占死亡总数的七分之一。这一数字在发达国家上升至四分之一到三分之一,那些地方因感染、营养不良或暴力导致的过早死亡风险相对要低得多。图1显示了世界不同地区确诊患癌的人数,图2和图3显示的是各个地区死于癌症的人数。各地区之间显然有很大的差别:世界某一地区很常见的癌症,在另一个地区却根本不在常见癌症之列。各列表中的差异实在太多,无法一一详细讨论。因此,我会介绍其中的一些例子,来说明为何存在这些差异,它们又是如何产生的。

肺 癌

在世界任何地方,肺癌都是癌症死亡的最大病因,这一类型的癌症致死数目占全部癌症死亡人数的17%,累计120万人。这是一种高度致命的疾病,在大多数国家,确诊此病的人的五年存活率还不到十分之一。就算在治疗结果最佳的美国,也只有不到五分之一的患者长期存活。此外,全世界的死亡率正在迅速升高,1975年到2002年间翻了一番。图1显示了全世界各种癌症的诊断率,清楚地表明肺癌是全球各地区的主要杀手之一。众所周知,吸烟与肺癌之间存在着强相关。因此,肺癌发病率的差异因吸烟率不同而不同也就不足为奇了。大多数情况下,肺癌在生命的相对后期才得到确诊,在大多数病例中都表现为超过半个世纪的大量吸烟(吸烟量较少的青年人群显然也会患上该病,但这类病例相对少见)。也就是说,肺癌的患病率以及该比率的趋势(上升还是下降)

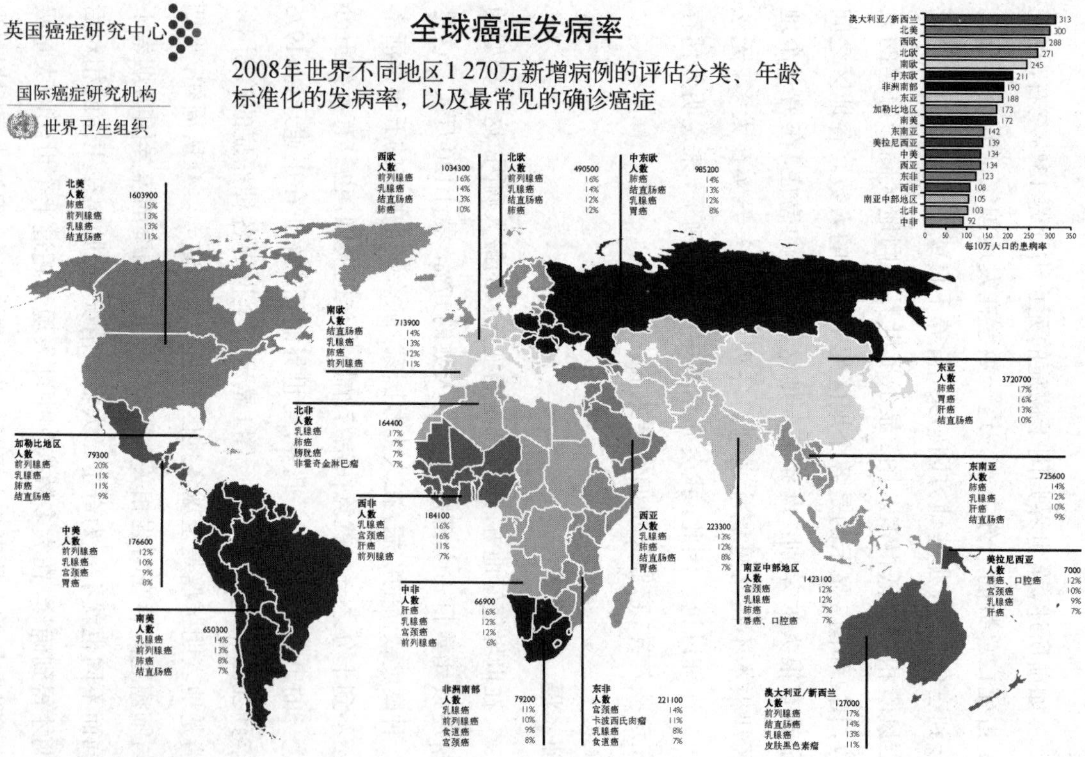

英国癌症研究中心
国际癌症研究机构
世界卫生组织
全球癌症发病率
2008年世界不同地区1 270万新增病例的评估分类、年龄标准化的发病率，以及最常见的确诊癌症
北美 人数 1603900 肺癌 15% 前列腺癌 13% 乳腺癌 13% 结直肠癌 11%
西欧 人数 1034300 前列腺癌 16% 乳腺癌 14% 结直肠癌 13% 肺癌 10%
北欧 人数 490500 前列腺癌 16% 乳腺癌 14% 结直肠癌 12% 肺癌 12%
中东欧 人数 985200 肺癌 14% 结直肠癌 13% 乳腺癌 12% 胃癌 8%
南欧 人数 713900 结直肠癌 14% 乳腺癌 13% 肺癌 12% 前列腺癌 11%
北非 人数 164400 乳腺癌 17% 肺癌 7% 膀胱癌 7% 非霍奇金淋巴瘤 7%
加勒比地区 人数 79300 前列腺癌 20% 乳腺癌 11% 肺癌 11% 结直肠癌 9%
中美 人数 176600 前列腺癌 12% 乳腺癌 10% 宫颈癌 9% 胃癌 8%
西非 人数 184100 乳腺癌 16% 宫颈癌 16% 肝癌 11% 前列腺癌 7%
西亚 人数 223300 乳腺癌 13% 肺癌 12% 结直肠癌 8% 胃癌 7%
中非 人数 66900 肝癌 16% 乳腺癌 12% 宫颈癌 12% 前列腺癌 6%
南美 人数 650300 乳腺癌 14% 前列腺癌 13% 肺癌 8% 结直肠癌 7%
非洲南部 人数 79200 乳腺癌 11% 前列腺癌 10% 食道癌 9% 宫颈癌 8%
东非 人数 221100 宫颈癌 14% 卡波西氏肉瘤 11% 乳腺癌 8% 食道癌 7%
东亚 人数 3720700 肺癌 17% 胃癌 16% 肝癌 13% 结直肠癌 10%
东南亚 人数 725600 肺癌 14% 乳腺癌 12% 肝癌 10% 结直肠癌 9%
南亚中部地区 人数 1423100 宫颈癌 12% 乳腺癌 12% 肺癌 7% 唇癌、口腔癌 7%
美拉尼西亚 人数 7000 唇癌、口腔癌 12% 宫颈癌 10% 乳腺癌 9% 肝癌 7%
澳大利亚/新西兰 人数 127000 前列腺癌 17% 结直肠癌 14% 乳腺癌 13% 皮肤黑色素瘤 11%
澳大利亚/新西兰 313
北美 300
西欧 288
北欧 271
南欧 245
中东欧 211
非洲南部 190
东亚 188
加勒比地区 173
南美 172
东南亚 142
美拉尼西亚 139
中美 134
西亚 134
东非 123
西非 108
南亚中部地区 105
北非 103
中非 92
0 50 100 150 200 250 300 350
每10万人口的患病率

图1 全球癌症发病率

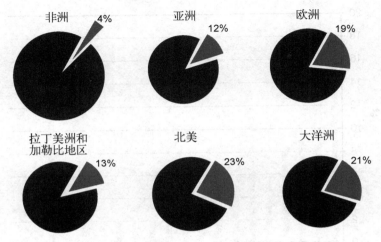

图 2　各大洲癌症死亡人数比例

反映了前半个世纪的吸烟习惯。如果我们知道了吸烟率的趋势，就可以预测某个人群肺癌患病率的未来趋势了。

在西欧和北美，男子吸烟率正呈下降之势，肺癌（以及与吸烟有关的其他疾病）的患病率也随之而落。与此相反，在发展中世界的大片地区，随着国家的工业化，吸烟率也迅速上升。日本的变化趋势就反映出这对癌症患病率的可能影响，1960—1980年间，在日本工业化的影响下，那里的肺癌患病率翻了不止一番。类似的变化如今在中国这样的国家也比较明显。原因有很多：在这些国家，吸烟这种习惯至今仍带着一种"酷炫"的光环，大大不同于烟民日益遭到唾弃的西方。那些国家的人们对与吸烟有关的健康问题意识一般较为淡薄，也没有实施在欧洲和北美日益常见的对烟草促销的限制。的确，在中国某个经济衰退的省份，官方近来还颁布命令，为了振兴当地的烟草种植业和提升税收，所有成年人都必须抽本地烟。因此，展望未来，我们会

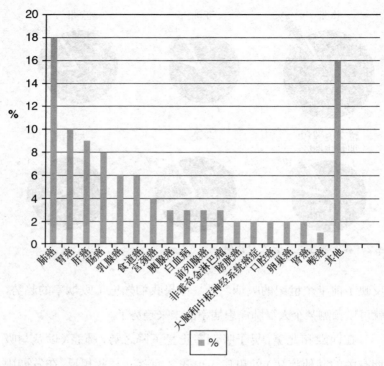

图3　全球癌症死因

发现，在"发达"世界的肺癌问题逐渐弱化的同时，新兴工业化国家将会面临日益增加的与吸烟有关的癌症（以及诸如心脏病等其他问题）的负担，除非它们迅速采纳如今西欧和北美常规的那些控烟策略。当前看来这不太可能，正在工业化的世界因而可能会披上发达世界那并不合意的外衣。

乳腺癌

从新增病例来看，乳腺癌是女性最常见的癌症，在女性癌症病例中占21%，在全球女性癌症死亡数量中占14%。不过，乳腺

8

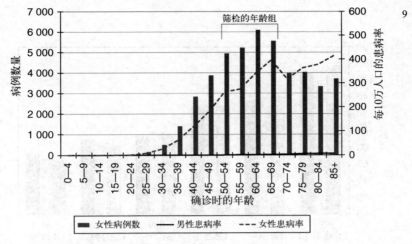

图4 2005年英国的乳腺癌诊断和死亡率

癌的整体存活率远胜肺癌，欧洲和北美有四分之三的患者能存活五年以上。就连欠发达国家也有过半数的乳腺癌患者实现了这一重要目标。

乳腺癌发生规律的研究也有助于表明，癌症统计数据在某些方面可以解释这种疾病的表现方式。

罹患乳腺癌的风险（与大多数癌症一样）随着年龄的增长而不断上升，从图4来自英国的数据就能看出这一点。所有发达国家都有着非常近似的分布。如果我们观察图中左侧的坐标轴——每个年龄段的实际患病人数——会发现峰值出现在50—70岁这一年龄段，虽然70岁以上年龄段的风险较高，但人数较少，因为死于其他原因的人数较多。还可以看到，尽管资金募集人常常在宣传材料中使用40岁以下女性的病例，这一年龄段的女性却鲜有确诊此病的。图5从另一个角度，即社会阶层的角度，考察了病例的分布。该图表明，较为富裕、受教育程度较高

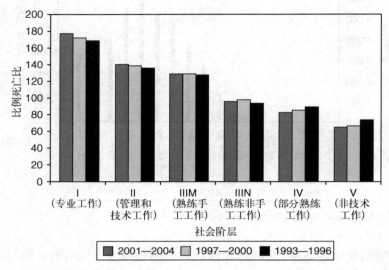

图 5　乳腺癌的诊断率和社会阶层

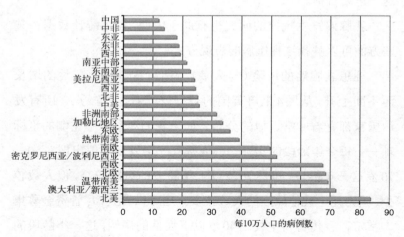

图 6　全世界乳腺癌诊断的差异

的女性罹患此病的风险明显高于不太宽裕的人。受过教育的中年女性往往是难以对付的社会运动参与者，既有时间，又有见识来有效地游说。就像我们在后文中将会看到的那样，癌症研究和治疗获得两者都不是纯粹根据需要来安排的，而往往会受到来自代表特殊群体的游说组织的巨大压力。

全世界乳腺癌风险诸图再次显示出一些惊人的趋势。图6明确指出，乳腺癌在某种程度上与富裕有关——富国的患病率高于穷国。至于烟草/癌症的关联，吸烟与风险之间有着十分明显的关系。我们很难理解，平均收入更高为何会增加某种疾病的风险——这与大多数公共卫生趋势背道而驰。那么原因是什么呢？一个因素是人口的年龄结构。正如图4所示，患癌的风险随着年龄而上升。因此，预期寿命短的贫穷国家女性或许只是因为寿命不够长而没来得及患上乳腺癌，在生命早期便已死于其他的疾病。然而，这并不能解释图中所示的风险在各年龄段的极大范围。对于观察到的潜在差异，有各种不同的理论，最可能的解释与激素对乳房组织的作用有关。例如，初次受孕年龄和怀孕次数对癌症风险有明显的影响。青春期开始时间晚、初孕时间早，以及怀孕频次较高看来都是预防乳腺癌的因素。在西方，因为营养较好和高蛋白饮食，青春期开始的时间比从前早，而因为有效的避孕、女性日趋独立以及更好的教育，怀孕发生得较晚。在贫穷国家，青春期来得较晚，女性对生育也缺乏控制。虽说这种情况显然会带来各种潜在的问题，看来却防止了乳腺癌。哺乳会在产后影响激素水平，似乎也能防止乳腺癌，目前西方受过良好教育的女性中更盛行哺乳，似乎可以预测趋势将向反方向倾斜。随着国家与个人收入的增加，出生率渐趋下

11

降,而初孕年龄却渐趋上升,因此可以预期,和肺癌一样,扩大发展将会导致全球乳腺癌病例的增加。

显然,乳房是终生随着激素水平变化(这是青春期、孕期、哺乳期、绝经期,或口服避孕药和激素替代疗法等药物治疗的结果)而变化的器官。从上述观察结果可以得出,影响激素水平的治疗或许可以改变罹患乳腺癌的风险。激素替代疗法(HRT)广泛用于绝经期症状。除了改善全身潮热和丧失性欲等症状之外,人们还希望HRT可以预防绝经期后日趋增多的疾病,诸如心脏病和会带来骨折风险的骨质流失(骨质疏松症)等。尽管HRT对于实现某些目标的确行之有效,但长期使用似乎又会增加乳腺癌的风险。口服避孕药片也一样,它也是通过改变正常的激素环境而起效的。因此,这些影响十分混乱:(与怀孕和哺乳关联的)某些激素变化可以防止乳腺癌,而(口服避孕药和HRT等)其他变化却会增加风险。有鉴于此,很多实验室研究都关注各种激素对于诱发乳腺癌所起的作用,以及研发通过干预激素的作用途径来治疗乳腺癌的药物。他莫昔芬正是这样的一种药物,它的主要功能是阻断雌激素的效用,可以被看作是有史以来最有效的药物之一,自进入临床应用以来,它在大约25年里拯救了足有数百万女性的生命,并帮助延长了更多人的寿命(见第三章)。

最后,有一种看法认为,乳腺癌是一种年轻女性的疾病,这种观念在某种程度上是由倡导更好治疗和研究的某些团体推动的。一般说来,正如我们已经看到的那样,这并不准确。然而,对乳腺癌风险模式的研究表明,某些家族罹患乳腺癌的风险似乎极高,母亲、姐妹、姨母都在早年染上此病,往往双侧患癌或伴随卵巢癌，男性亲属也会患上前列腺癌。这些家族显然是深入研究的理想对象，鉴于这些家族的风险如此明显，患者往往会非常愿意参与研究。对这类病例的遗传模式的研究表明，乳腺癌的风险从母亲传给孩子的可能性是50%，并提出这种疾病至少有两种常见的遗传形式，外加一系列不太常见的形式。第二章对这个研究领域有更详细的说明。

肝 癌

肝癌是全世界最常见的癌症之一，但它的分布模式与肺癌和乳腺癌大不相同。让人感兴趣的是，一种可以免费注射的（乙型肝炎）疫苗接种可以有效预防患上肝癌。总体而言，以新增病例来说，它是第六常见的癌症，但在导致死亡的癌症中却是第三常见的死因，表明这种疾病极为凶险。肝癌病例模式中有不少关键特征值得更详细的考察。中国和非洲部分地区的发病率比欧洲和北美高出五至七倍。这种疾病几乎是致命的，部分原因在于它发生在公共卫生欠发达的地区，但主要原因是乙肝病毒（HBV）会对肝脏造成严重伤害，从而导致了这种疾病。

肝癌与肝脏的长期受损有关，在欧洲和北美，这通常是酗酒造成的。在这种癌症更常见的世界某些地区，更重要的病因是 HBV 感染。1965年，巴鲁克·布隆伯格博士首次描述了这种情况，并为此获颁诺贝尔奖。多年以前，流行病学研究就确定了肝炎与肝癌之间的联系。后续的研究发现，病毒的分子生物学同样表明它有着直接致病作用，而不是偶然关联。在建立了病毒和癌症之间的联系后，治疗一种常见癌症的疫苗就切实可行了。令所有相关人士大感宽慰的是，HBV 疫苗接种大获成功，风险最

13

高的人群迅速获益。

消化道癌

一般来说,消化道癌要么发生在顶端(胃和食道),要么发生在末端(结肠和直肠),中段(小肠)的癌症相对罕见。消化道癌的模式有一些有趣的趋势,我会一一道来,先从顶端的胃癌开始。

总体而言,每年几乎有100万人确诊胃癌,其中有大约三分之二被这种疾病折磨致死——至少有65万人之众。如图7所示,过去50年来,西方的胃癌发病率持续下降,过去它是一种相对常见的癌症,如今则相当罕见。在世界其他地区,胃癌发病率也开始下降了,但时间较为晚近。人们提出了各种可能原因,从价格低廉的冰箱的普及到胃溃疡的治疗,但确切的原因目前尚未完全查清。

大肠的各种癌症也表明人群之间存在巨大的差异。大体上说,大肠癌在欧洲和北美很常见,在远东就不太常见了,在非洲则很罕见。因此,这主要是一种发达世界的疾病。总的来说,每年约有100万人确诊此病,其中大约一半患者因此而死亡。如今由于认识提高、早期诊断和疗效改善,该病在北美和欧洲的死亡率呈下降之势。对移民的研究表明,这种差异与环境有关,无关种族——从低风险国家移民到高风险国家的人会迅速呈现出新家园的风险模式。此外,在日本等日益采纳西化饮食的国家,该病的发病率则有所上升。因此,这种结果的主要可能原因是饮食——低位肠道内壁环境的差异显然来自顶端进食之物的差别!如此说来,似乎存在着某种交互影响——过去50年来饮食的变化让胃癌日益罕见,却导致肠道另一端患癌的风险增加。

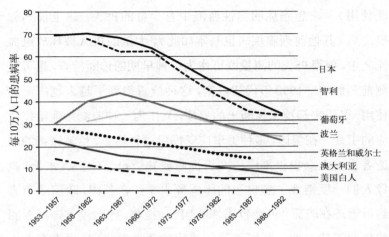

图7 过去若干年来的胃癌患病率

研究这类变化给各种癌症的起源提供了重要的线索，同时还可以为发现预防策略指明方向。

前列腺癌

　　前列腺癌是一种有趣的疾病。在欧洲和北美，它是男性最常确诊的癌症，也是男性的主要癌症死因之一。2007年，全球有67万男性确诊此病。致死率难以确定，因为确诊患有早期前列腺癌的很多男性并非死于这种疾病。和乳腺癌一样，不同国家之间的死亡率差异很大。某些差异似乎是前列腺特异抗原（PSA）血检应用率的差异造成的，这种检查能够发现早期癌症，可以作为一种筛检。

　　PSA是前列腺产生的一种蛋白质，其正常功能是液化射精期间产生的液体（题外话——啮齿动物没有PSA，它们在交配期间会产生一种固体的精液栓，而小鼠却在前列腺癌研究中被广泛使用）。未患癌症的男性血液中有少量的PSA。患上前列腺癌之后（其他前列腺疾病也基本如此），大量的PSA被释放进血流之中，使得PSA的测量既可作为一种早期的诊断检查，也可监测前列腺癌。1990年代初以来，这种检查得到了越来越广泛的使用，既用来筛检未诊断出的癌症，又作为一种监测癌症治疗反应的工具。在美国，多种渠道广泛提供这种检查，检测试剂的制造者也向大众积极推广——男性需要知道自己的PSA水平，就像人们一度需要了解自己的胆固醇水平。在英国，政府政策直到最近还在阻碍"机会致病性的"PSA检测，因为没有证据表明前列腺癌的早期诊断能够降低该病的死亡率，所以也没有出台全面的筛检计划。近来的筛检试验数据表明，PSA检测或许可以降低前列腺癌的死亡率，但在大约40个由PSA检测发现而得到治疗的男性中，只有一人能免于死亡。这种获益水平是否会促使政府确立筛检计划仍有待观察。应当指出，乳腺癌筛检的获益水平也差不多，只是人们把它想象得很高，所以乳腺癌筛检在整个西方世界被极为广泛地使用，而PSA筛检虽然得到了广泛应用，其好处却远不及前者鲜明。目前，全世界的PSA筛检差别很大，大体上是由消费者推动的。

如果从前列腺癌的诊断和死亡率开始考察，我们可以看到某些非常明显的差异（图8）。欧洲人和北美人比居住在中南半岛的男性的死亡率要高得多，后者患上此病相对罕见，在非洲大部分地区也是一样。欧洲和北美内部还有更多有趣的差异，距离赤道越远，死亡率就越高，这在美国和澳大利亚的白种人之间最为明显，这两地白人人口的种族特征相当一致。如果我们观察种族影响，也会发现惊人的差别：非裔男性的前列腺癌死亡率大约是白种人的两倍。与此相反，中南半岛裔保持了其来源地区的较低风险，这和在女性与乳腺癌中所观察到的结果相近。

该如何解释这种情况？最佳证据表明，白种人和亚裔族群之间的差异，是饮食的差异外加对引发前列腺癌的无论何种因素（这基本上还不得而知）的种族敏感性差异所导致的。纬度的差别更难以用饮食来解释，显然也不能用种族来解释，因为欧洲、北美和澳大利亚均有病例。最好的解释似乎是日晒，日晒是有保护作用的。鉴于目前各种大型公共健康运动都提倡人们减少日晒，这不啻是个非常惊人的结论。日晒怎么会影响某个内脏器官的患癌风险？要知道这个内脏可是最"不会见光"的啊。答案似乎是维生素D。缺乏维生素D会导致佝偻病，令人想起维多利亚时期的济贫院和畸形的儿童，但这种疾病或许相当于21世纪癌症风险的上升，以下文字框对此做出了总结。

维生素D、阳光与癌症

维生素D密切参与了大量组织的生长和发育，其中就包括前列腺和乳房等腺体结构。维生素D的新陈代谢相当复杂，但关键的一步是在皮肤中发生的，且需要阳光。长期缺乏日晒可能会导致"活性"维生素D的缺乏——这倒还不足以引发佝偻病，却足以略微改变患上前列腺癌的概率。这还可以解释为何通常肤色最暗的非裔男性如果住在温带地区，患上前列腺癌的风险最高。如果这个假设是正确的，就可以预测在人群中日晒时间最长的白种人患上前列腺癌的风险较低。皮肤癌是个衡量日晒的好指标，已有人对皮肤癌患者的前列腺癌风险进行了研究。正如预测的那样，由皮肤损伤和皮肤癌证明的日晒时间最长的人，其患上前列腺癌的风险降低了。此外，日晒增加之后，个体患上前列腺癌的风险有很大的下降——一项研究估计，会降低40%之多。就连那些处于前列腺癌发展期的人，日晒似乎也会显著延缓确诊——日晒时间最短的人确诊的平均年龄为67岁，日晒时间最长的为72岁，延缓了大约5年之久。因此，核心思想看来非常一致——男性群体的最大杀手可以通过更多的日光浴来预防，然而公共卫生政策的建议却反对这样做！

如果前列腺癌存在这种影响，并显然受到了皮肤中产生的循环因子的调节，那么在其他癌症中能否也见到这种情况？答案看来是肯定的，而且这种影响的大小在几乎所有内脏癌症中似乎没有多大差别。随日晒增加而导致风险上升的唯一一类癌症就是皮肤癌（特别是黑色素瘤），事实上死于这种癌症的人数相对极少。因此，对前列腺癌死亡率的研究揭示了各种关于常见癌症病因的有趣内容，并抛出一种非常惊人的关联，从根本上挑战了当前标准的公共卫生建议。在作者看来，关于日晒的既定认知亟须彻底更正。

在诊断和死亡率方面还有第二组惊人的差异。比方说，如果我们比较英国和美国，就会看到每10万人口的死亡率非常接近，但诊断率大不相同，美国前列腺癌诊断率与死亡率之比是英国的两倍以上。从另一个角度来看，美国前列腺癌患者的死亡率远低于英国。

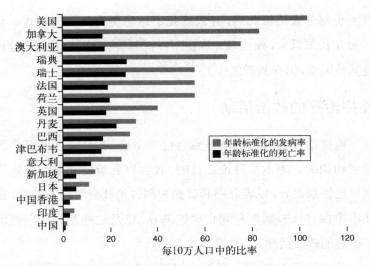

图8 前列腺癌的发病率和死亡率

这有若干可能的解释——在美国,前列腺癌或许真的要常见得多,以及美国的医疗系统治疗此病比英国系统要好两倍。尽管与美国医疗系统相比,英国系统的治疗结果确实略逊一筹,但对于大多数癌症来说,这些差异只是几个百分点的差距,不大可能解释治愈率的明显差距。此外,考察一下其他常见癌症的检测率,就会发现英美两国每10万人口的检出率大致相近,这说明有其他因素在起作用。答案就在于PSA血检。

公共政策的差别以及PSA检测的普及度导致英国接受检查的男性人数远低于美国,因而该病的诊断率也要低得多。然而,美国的PSA血检率高,而确诊此病的大多数美国人病情的临床表现轻微。如果不是确诊此病,他们大概不会被它困扰,这表明之所以会存在发病率的巨大差异,大体上是因为跟英国相比,美国对相对并不致命的轻度疾病的诊断率较高。大西洋两岸都

19

有一小部分人确诊此病，并最终死于该病更为凶险的形式。从1990年代末以来，死亡率一直在下降，但这应直接归因于筛检还是其他因素，仍在激辩之中。

癌症治疗的政治活动

癌症治疗的政治活动显然有很多角度，都与该病的经济因素密切相关。为本章讨论之目的，我会以乳腺癌和前列腺癌为例讨论性别差异，以乳腺癌和肺癌为例讨论社会阶层的影响，由此集中探讨诊断病例和死亡率的差异，以及这些差异如何推动了该病的政治活动。

前列腺癌在很多方面都可以说是与乳腺癌对应的男性疾病。它们的相似性可以延伸到很多层面：两个器官在性行为和生殖方面都起到了一定的作用；两者都会根据激素水平而终生发生变化；两种癌症都可通过改变激素环境来治疗；而治疗两个器官各自发生的癌症均会导致性功能的深刻变化。在政治上，数十年来，乳房那强有力的性象征及情感意象，一直被用于将大量研究和治疗资金引入乳腺癌，效果极其明显。这使得女性乳腺癌病患的结果得到了稳定的逐步改善，具体体现为存活率提高了，成功治疗所造成的损伤也有所减少。例如，越来越多的女性接受了伤残程度较低的手术或乳房重建，而不是激进的乳房切除术。在药物资金问题上，女性也一直在卓有成效地争取新的治疗方法——曲妥珠单抗（又被称为"赫赛汀"）在整个欧洲和北美医疗系统中的迅速应用就是证明。

直到最近，尽管两种癌症在生物学上可以分庭抗礼，却没有类似的运动来支持男性前列腺癌患者，也没有旨在改善治疗和效

癌症

果的倡议出现。例如，截至1995年，英国在前列腺癌研究上的开销只有乳腺癌的十分之一。过去十年间，情况有所改变，部分原因就在于PSA检测。这使得前列腺癌的种种情况大幅"左倾"，晚期病例减少，早期病例增多，治疗的选择也更加多样，并且该病有了治愈的可能，带病存活期也延长了。鉴于政治和经济权力大都集中在中老年男人手中——他们最有可能患上这种疾病，却鲜有患上乳腺癌的（尽管男人也会患上此病）——历史上一贯缺乏对前列腺癌的公共卫生和研究兴趣便尤其令人惊讶。究其根本原因，差别似乎来自男人和女人不同的心理——女人谈论乳腺癌实属平常，谈论乳腺癌的女人并不会被视为弱者，往往还会被视为自强不息的典范，凯莉·米洛①近来的全球巡回演唱会便是一例。另一方面，在以前男人们对这种疾病感到非常难以启齿，特别是在治疗附带着诸如阳痿和失禁等"无男子气概"的风险时，更不要提诊断所需的途径（通过直肠）在本质上便令人尴尬不已。加之大多数男人在与健康有关的所有事情上普遍采取"鸵鸟"态度，结果便是男人要付出寿命较短、不及女人健康的代价。

然而，公共和经济政策近来发生了变化，为男性治疗和研究该病投入的资金增加了。部分程度上，这无疑是由于制药业终于意识到，针对这一西方世界最大的男性癌症杀手的投入，利润空间不可限量。科林·鲍威尔、罗杰·摩尔和鲁道夫·朱利安尼等重要公众人物的态度也发生了变化，他们开始愿意公开谈论自己接受该病治疗的情况了。

---

① 凯莉·米洛（1968— ），澳洲歌手、作曲家、演员。2005年，凯莉被诊断罹患乳腺癌。2006年末康复后，她重返乐坛，随后展开了全球巡回演唱会。

最后，在癌症治疗政治活动这一背景下，吸烟和公共政策的问题也值得一提，因为在过去的几十年里，这个问题在世界各地差异很大。不久前，烟草公司实际上还在投放这样的广告标语，说某种香烟是医生们偏爱的品牌。吸烟与各种癌症风险增加之间的关联是流行病学研究的成就之一，使得发达世界吸烟率和与之相关的各种疾病的患病率大幅下降。促成这一结果的有一系列措施，从立法（禁烟）到教育（禁止广告和赞助，健康警示语），再到财政（对该商品征税，这是额外的收益，可用于给吸烟者收拾残局，支付所需的医疗费用）。然而，发展中世界的情况不同：吸烟仍被认为很"酷"，针对年轻人的广告和营销也支持这种暗示，而在欧洲和北美，越来越多的人认为抽烟是遭人唾弃的行为，只配在寒冷的大门外进行。此外，大型跨国烟草公司在把金钱带给发展中国家的同时，也拥有了强大的政治影响力，可用于缓和公共卫生对这种习惯的口诛笔伐（西方世界就曾抨击声不断）。再加上发展中国家年轻的人口结构，发展中世界与吸烟相关的癌症——肺癌、膀胱癌、咽喉癌、口腔癌——将在未来几年流行开来。在中国这样迅速现代化、生活标准提高、预期寿命延长的国家，预计这将导致这些癌症的发病率大幅增加。

第二章

癌症的发展

为理解癌症的发展，有必要了解一点细胞生物学的基础知识。细胞是所有生物的基本组成部分。从酵母菌这种最微小的生物到最庞大的蓝鲸，全都由细胞组成，人体也一样。某些动物——如酵母菌——是单细胞的；包括我们在内的其他动物都是由不同类别的很多细胞组成的，包括血液、骨骼、大脑、肾脏，诸如此类。有机体的所有细胞都有其精心控制的生命周期。该周期的控制一旦出现问题，癌症就发生了，导致一群细胞不受控制地生长，它们可以扩散到体内的其他结构并造成破坏。本章重点讨论癌症的发展，以及理解这一历程所需的基础生物学知识。我还会阐述对于病因的理解是如何能够用来确定治疗策略的。

就理解肿瘤①而言，细胞的关键部分是细胞核，那里有包含基因密码的脱氧核糖核酸（DNA）。图9是DNA分子的示意图。

_____

① 结合语境此处将"cancer"翻译为临床上常用的"肿瘤"，特指癌症的生理表现。下文同。——编注

DNA受损导致异常的、不受控制的细胞生长，这是肿瘤发生的根本原因。值得注意的是，尽管不同细胞的外观和功能或许迥然不同（例如神经细胞、肌肉细胞以及血细胞等），特定有机体内的所有细胞却共享着相同的DNA密码。DNA聚集而成的长链被称为染色体，每个人类细胞里都有23对染色体。在每条染色体中，基因排布在DNA上，每个基因编码产生一种蛋白质。我们可以把基因和染色体想象成一座图书馆，23对染色体中的每一对都是一个独立的卷册，21 000个基因中的每一个都是该卷册中的一页说明书。在概念上很容易理解一页说明书的损坏何以导致细胞性状的改变。本章将历数这些不同结构的功能和相互作用，以及它们何以出错，从而导致某种肿瘤的发展。

　　每个人的生命都始自一颗受精卵，它首先发育成一团相同的细胞，然后逐渐生长、编组、发育成一个完整的复杂个体。细胞从这个初始的群组发育成高度专门化的亚型的过程是大自然最绝妙的复杂过程之一，但它却在我们的周围和体内不断发生。这显然需要一个错综复杂的制衡网络。它需要相邻细胞之间的交流，以确保在适当的时间遵循正确的发育路径。它需要以最少的中断来清理和消除不再需要的细胞[这个过程称作细胞凋亡（apoptosis），源自希腊语，意为"花瓣的脱落"]。随着器官的发育，它们必须发展自己的血液供应并加以维护，以应对损伤。它需要各器官系统彼此交流，例如神经要与它们所控制的肌肉联系。内分泌（激素）腺体要加以协调，才能周期性（如卵巢）或是应激性（如肾上腺）地产生其产物。这是随着每个器官系统的生长和发育，以协同的方式通过基因的打开或关闭来实现的。一旦生长过程结束，动物成形，就必须维持各个组织，修复

损伤，并持续综合管理——供应和加工养分，清除废物，如此等
等。我们越是思考所有这些任务令人叹为观止的复杂度，就越
是感叹此事非同寻常：整个过程在大多数人身上如此可靠地运
作了这么多年，而肿瘤——从本质上说就是不受管制的细胞分
裂——的发生频率却并未升高。

DNA 的结构和功能

如上所述，遗传密码储存在人体细胞的23对染色体里。每
一条染色体都由一个很长的DNA分子组成，其中包含着基因，
点缀着间隔序列。每个基因的两侧都是DNA区域，控制某个特
定基因的开启或关闭。例如，肌肉细胞的关键组分肌凝蛋白的
基因编码会在需要的地方——肌肉中——开启，在其他不需要
它的组织比如神经细胞中关闭。开关网络显然对于调控细胞行
为非常关键，对这些控制的研究是癌症研究的主要内容——如
果控制失灵，细胞就会毫无节制地生长，肿瘤发生时就是如此。

为了理解细胞如何行使所有这些功能，有必要多了解一点
DNA的结构，以及嵌在DNA分子中的密码如何被翻译为最终产
物，即功能有机体。DNA是脱氧核糖核酸的缩写。1953年，克
里克和沃森发现了DNA的双螺旋结构，早在这一著名的发现之
前，人们就已经知道它含有遗传密码了。DNA分子（图9所示）
是交互排列的两个组件所形成的一条长脊，这两个组件分别是
一种糖（称作脱氧核糖）和一种磷酸基团，后者连接着腺嘌呤、
鸟嘌呤、胞嘧啶和胸腺嘧啶四种所谓的碱基分子（简称A、G、C、
T）。这些碱基沿着DNA分子的脊排列，形成了A-T和C-G相
互连接的两组互补配对。DNA的双螺旋性质来自（正链或正意

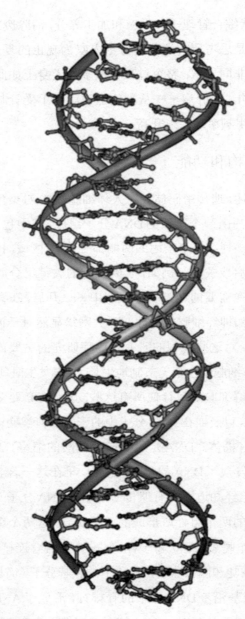

图 9 DNA 的结构

的）一股和与之互补的反意股相匹配，A 与 T 配对，C 与 G 配对，
以此类推。如此一来，A–T 对和 C–G 对就构成了维持 DNA 双链
的双螺旋结构的"胶水"。结合过程的互补性质意味着如果把
两条链分开，每条链都用作两组新链的模板，就能得到与起初那
个 DNA 分子完全相同的两个副本。

　　DNA 可以制造与自身完全相同的副本这种固有性质，是地
球上所有生命的基本特性之一。从最简单到最复杂的，所有生
命都非常严格地保留了 DNA 的结构。复制过程同样极其精确。
错误率如此之低，以至于需要很多世代才能累积出显著的差
异——遗传"漂变"率——这也是演化生物学的基础之一。回
到遗传学的"图书馆藏书"这个比喻上来：细胞每一次分裂，都
必须把全部 23 对各卷册以及其中的 21 000 个基因（信息的"书
页"）"逐字"记录。有时，一个逗号、字母或句号会发生打字错
误。在大多数情况下，就像在书中一样，这种错误不会改变意
义，但有时会发生重大改变，从而导致子细胞携带了改变（称作
突变）后的功能。顺便提一下，随机的微小差异数量可以在进化
树上追查，如此便可估计某一对特定的物种是何时开始分化的。

基因，以及基因表达的控制

　　基因是组成 DNA 的基本单位。一个基因包含了一种蛋白
质的密码。蛋白质可以具有多种功能，从结构性的功能，例如一
种构成细胞内部"骨架"的名为微管蛋白的蛋白质，到运作性的
功能，例如形成可收缩的肌肉的部分。DNA 中的信息借以转录
为一种（RNA 里的）讯息，随后转录到某种单一的蛋白质之中，
这一信息流正是生物学的核心概念之一。

蛋白质是细胞的重要组件，负责所有的重要活动。诸如脂类和糖类等其他构件都是作为蛋白质活动的结果而生成的。因此，蛋白质显然必须具有一系列的功能。这些功能包括：在细胞内部和细胞间传送信号；充当结构（一种微观的脚手架）；以及有一种非常重要的蛋白质——酶，这种蛋白质作用于其他的生物分子，促使新分子的形成。这个过程可以是毁灭性的，比如分解食物的消化道分泌物（以及洗衣粉！）中的酶；也可以是建设性的，比如参与为细胞制造新分子的酶。

基因产生蛋白质的过程涉及基因转录成细胞核内的一种信使核糖核酸（mRNA）分子。RNA分子的结构与DNA相似，但在关键方面有所不同。首先，主链中的脱氧核糖（DNA中的D）被核糖（RNA中的R）所代替。其次，该分子是单链的。最后，胸腺嘧啶（T）碱基被尿嘧啶（U）所代替，但配对保持不变。

为了制造RNA，DNA的双螺旋临时"解开"形成两条单独的链。随后组装出一个互补RNA并将其运出细胞核，进入细胞质，DNA链再次合上。这个过程被称作转录（如图10所示），是生物学的另一个重要部分。

一旦进入细胞质，这个信使RNA就必须被转化成蛋白质，这是嵌在DNA中的密码被翻译成功能性蛋白质的第二个重要部分。第二种RNA——称作转运RNA——提供了信使RNA和蛋白质构件之间的联系。这个翻译过程的关键之处在于嵌在DNA中的三联体密码。蛋白质和DNA一样，都是由更简单的分子链组成的。蛋白质的构件被称作氨基酸，可以连在一起，形成实际上无穷无尽的长链。基本的氨基酸分子有三个要素——被

29

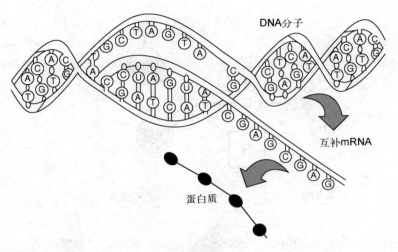

图10　转录

称为羧基端和氨基端（因此得名），加上赋予每一种氨基酸其独特性质的可变侧支（图11中表示为R）。

　　尽管理论上存在无穷数量的氨基酸，但在活的生物体中只找到了20种。DNA密码是以名为密码子的三联体排列的。A、T/U、C和G可以组成64种可能的三字母密码。每一个三联体都有特定的含义，既可以指代一种氨基酸，也可以实际上形成一种标点符号。例如，在这个密码系统中，AUG的意思是"从这里开始"（称作"起始密码子"）；UAG、UGA和UAA的意思是"在这里结束"；其余的部分都与特定氨基酸有关联——例如，半胱氨酸是UGU或UGC。因为三联体密码有64种可能的组合，却只有20种氨基酸，所以某些氨基酸有不止一个三联体密码。因此，显而易见，改变了单个碱基的突变可以从根本上改变最终的蛋白质。例如，从UGC（半胱氨酸）变成UGA（停止信号）会让最 30
终得到的蛋白质变短，其功能也可能发生重大的变化。

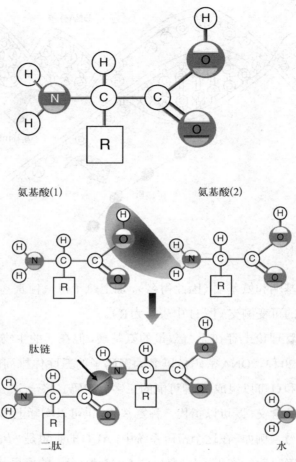

氨基酸(1)　　　　　　　　　　氨基酸(2)

肽链

二肽　　　　　　　　　　　　　水

图11　氨基酸与蛋白质的结构

　　如上所述，基因的核心密码伴随着复杂的调节机制（见图12）以确保基因在适当的时间开合。在癌细胞里，往往正是这种基因功能调节机制出现了缺陷。

　　基因表达的调节需要一系列复杂事件的相互作用。为了理解这一点，我们需要更详细地了解一下基因结构（见图12）。

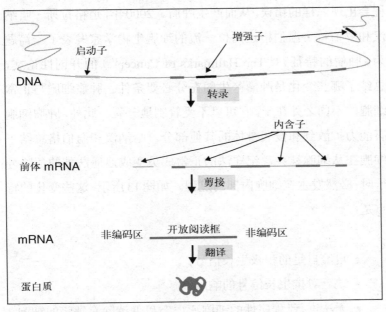

图 12　基因的结构与功能

基因编码区域的两侧是控制区。正如前文讨论过的编码区突变那样，基因调节或信使 RNA 的加工所发生的变化如何导致了某种蛋白质过度生成或生成不足，或是产生了带有某种不良性质的异常蛋白质，就很容易理解了。这些控制区域本身也受到名为转录因子的其他基因的调节，这些转录因子可以像控制音量一样提高和降低基因的表达。转录因子是整个过程的主要调节者，因此涉及肿瘤的很多基因事实上都来自这一族蛋白质，也就不足为奇了。

肿瘤的特征

介绍完这个机制的基础知识后，我们现在就来看看这些过

32

程会出现怎样的错误，从而产生肿瘤。2000年，道格拉斯·哈纳汉和罗伯特·温伯格这两位一流的细胞生物学家发表了一篇题为《肿瘤的特征》（"The Hallmarks of Cancer"）的开创性论文，总结了哪些变化是肿瘤产生的充分必要条件。肿瘤细胞与正常细胞的不同之处在于，它可以不受管制地分裂。此外，肿瘤细胞有能力扩散到和侵袭身体的其他部分。哈纳汉和温伯格总结了细胞在从细胞社会遵纪守法的正常成员变成逍遥法外的危险分子时，必然发生在细胞内部的过程。如图13所示，这些变化的特点是：

- 自给自足的积极生长信号；
- 缺乏对抗生长信号的响应；
- 无法进行"程序性的细胞死亡"，以便清除有缺陷的细胞；
- 规避免疫系统的破坏；
- 能够在其他组织中生长并破坏性地侵袭后者；
- 能够通过产生新的血管来维持生长。

前两个特点算是不言自明，并导致了不受管制的生长。第三个就不那么明显了，它与发育过程有关。如果所有的细胞都只是生长和分裂，举例而言，那就绝无可能形成诸如消化道或血管这样的中空管道结构了。为了做到这一点，根据结构发育的需求，必须把某些细胞清除出正在生长的有机体。前面提到过，这个过程被称为细胞凋亡，是一个重要的细胞功能。细胞凋亡也是有机体用来摆脱有缺陷或功能异常细胞的手段，例如那些寿限将至、需要替换的细胞。肿瘤细胞顾名思义是异常细胞，所以

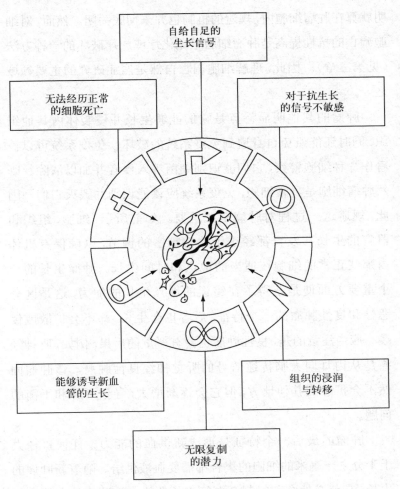

图 13 肿瘤的特征

本应自行了断。如此说来，无法进行细胞凋亡是从异常细胞转
变为能够无限复制的细胞的关键。细胞凋亡的另一个特点是，33
被化学疗法或放射疗法损伤的细胞常常不是当场死亡，而仅仅
是"身负重伤"。随后的细胞死亡往往是由细胞凋亡实现的，表

明就算在肿瘤细胞内，规避的机制也并未彻底关闭。然而，对细胞凋亡的抗性提高是肿瘤细胞避免化疗或放疗破坏的一种方法（见第三章）。因此，理解细胞凋亡自然是癌症研究的主要领域之一。

肿瘤的其他明显特点是它们能够生长并侵袭体内其他组织，同时还能避免自身遭到免疫系统的破坏。免疫系统可以被看作一种细胞警察，它们能识别细菌等入侵者并加以清除。既然肿瘤细胞是异常细胞，免疫系统应该能识别并毁灭它们。因此，规避这一过程对肿瘤至关重要。如前所示，细胞、组织和器官的生长和发育都经过了非常精密的调节，以确保有机体内那些正常的细胞在适当的地点和时间生长。肿瘤生长的一个重要方面便是获得了在错误的地点生长的能力，这是区分恶性和良性肿瘤的一个特征，后者也会生长，却不会扩散或侵袭。应当注意的是，良性肿瘤也会有严重的后果，例如，听神经瘤是从内耳向大脑传递信号的听觉神经良性肿瘤。该肿瘤固然不会扩散到其他地方，但它会逐渐增大，导致耳聋和平衡的问题。

肿瘤的最后一个特征是形成新供血的能力。任何直径大于十分之一毫米的细胞的集合都需要血液供给。随着新肿瘤的生长，它就必然会获得刺激血管生长的能力。肿瘤的血管生长往往杂乱无章，事实上它使用的是与维护正常血管无关的基因。这个过程被称为肿瘤的血管形成，因为它不同于正常的血管形成，所以成为肿瘤药物开发的一个重要的靶子。如果有可能破坏肿瘤的供血，就可以阻止它继续生长。贝伐珠单抗（安维汀）

是新一代靶向分子疗法中最成功的药物之一，就是针对这个过程来发挥作用的。

癌变——癌症是如何开始的

如前所示，如果发生了肿瘤的特征所需的那些变化，就会导致癌症。为了理解癌症的发展，我们现在要谈一谈外部因素是如何引发癌症的——这个过程被称为癌变。从本质上说，肿瘤是DNA受损的结果，从而导致了上文所述以及图13所示的变化。因此，所有破坏DNA的因子都是潜在的致癌物，即导致癌症的诱因。但反之则不然；本身有助于致癌的因子并不一定会直接破坏DNA，尽管在这个过程结束时总是如此。并非直接破坏DNA的致癌物质的例子包括酒精，以及会引发乳腺癌和前列腺癌的性激素等。致癌物有很多种，其中一些是众所周知的——例如吸烟和电离辐射。以吸烟为例，我们知道，在一般情况下，吸烟多年才会导致癌症发展。这表明癌变过程既缓慢又可能有多个步骤。我们从前文的讨论可以预测，必然有多组基因发生突变，才会导致哈纳汉和温伯格描述的标志性变化。这一事件链也是在1990年代初提出的，如今往往称之为"福格尔斯泰因级联"，链条上的每一步都代表了一个新的突变（图14）。

福格尔斯泰因博士的小组研究了遗传性肠癌，在这种癌症的患者身上可以识别出一些公认的癌前（又称恶性肿瘤前）阶段。他们从患者身上采集了一些组织，着手识别在从正常的肠道内膜到临床上明显的肿瘤这一路径上，哪些基因在这许多阶段中发生了异常。结果证明，对于级联中每个阶段的发生，所需破坏的候选基因都是可以识别出来的。后续工作表明，尽管具

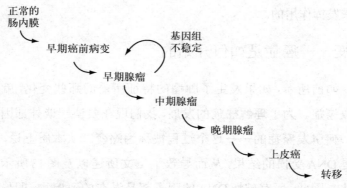

正常的
肠内膜

早期癌前病变

基因组
不稳定

早期腺瘤

中期腺瘤

晚期腺瘤

上皮癌

转移

图14　福格尔斯泰因级联

体的基因和破坏的次序不同，但类似的事件级联适用于所有的
肿瘤类型。

　　研究患有所谓"遗传性"癌症的家族，是识别基因的一种富
有成效的方式。这个术语不太恰当，因为癌症可不是钻石项链
之类的传家宝，也就是说，它不能作为一个原封未动、完好无损
的物件传承下去。所遗传的是某种疾病在生命早期发展起来的
高风险，这种疾病往往以非常夸张、极具侵袭性的形式爆发。有
一种这样的疾病叫腺瘤性结肠息肉（APC）。此病的患者从幼
年便开始长出多个良性肿瘤。一段时间以后，某些良性肿瘤发
展成癌症，不加治疗的话，一般会在40岁出头死于肠癌。对该病
患者的研究表明，他们的一个特定的基因出现了异常，该基因被
命名为APC。识别这些患者体内的APC基因引发对该基因功
能的进一步研究，证明它的功能就像一个"关闭键"。如果该基
因失去效能，就移除了细胞生长的一个重要制约，腺瘤也就形成
了。与遗传性癌症通常出现的方式一样，更加常见的非遗传性
癌症也有相似的异常情况。对非遗传性肠癌的研究证实，这些

散发的病例中，APC基因功能失效的约占80%，因此，该基因显然在调节肠道内膜的正常生长方面起到了关键的作用。

于是，对遗传性癌症的研究往往会为非遗传性的对应疾病提供重要的线索。对这些"癌症家族"的研究有助于识别像APC、Rb（与一种罕见的儿童眼部肿瘤——视网膜母细胞瘤有关）、p53（与李–佛美尼综合征①有关，该病患者会发展出多种不同的肿瘤），以及VHL（与一种包括肾癌在内的复杂疾病冯希佩尔–林道综合征②有关）这些与癌症有关的关键基因。此外，考察遗传性疾病各不相同的自然历史，有助于我们理解这些基因的正常功能应该是什么。上述的所有基因都被称为"肿瘤抑制者"基因，但这个词并不恰当，因为这并非它们在有机体内的主要作用。从APC基因便可预测，这些基因都是细胞周期的关键调节者（上文提到的前两个特征），功能的破坏或消除会导致不受控的生长。考察这些基因的正常功能为了解细胞周期的调节提供了重要的线索。正如缺乏对细胞周期的控制是肿瘤的一个特征，很多癌症治疗都是通过干预在肿瘤细胞内哑火的细胞周期基因起效的。此外，新一代癌症药物——靶向分子疗法——目前正进入临床阶段，成为新闻头条（见第三章）。这些药物之所以有效，正是因为它们针对的是已知在肿瘤中会哑火的特定分子。

然而，并不是遗传性癌症的所有基因都会直接参与细胞周期。一个很好的例子就是VHL基因，它最初是在冯希佩尔–林

---

① 一种罕见的自体显性遗传疾病。

② 又名家族性小脑视网膜血管瘤病，是一种罕见的常染色体显性遗传性疾病，表现为血管母细胞瘤累及小脑、脊髓、肾脏以及视网膜。

道综合征患者身上识别出来的。患者在幼年便出现多种异常病症，包括神经系统的囊肿，特别是在小脑（大脑中负责平衡和协调的部分）、脊髓和视网膜中，同时伴随良性和恶性的肾脏肿瘤。肾脏肿瘤通常是对称多发的，并且发生自幼年。至于APC，患者会遗传到一个无功能的基因；对余下基因的一次打击便可让细胞内再没有能够发挥作用的VHL蛋白质。肾脏肿瘤相对罕见，但在VHL综合征患者中很常见，这告诉我们，某种特定基因遭受一次打击的概率相当高，但遭受两次打击的间隔却要长得多，因此，散发肿瘤都是单独出现的，且发病的年龄晚得多。

对VHL基因的详细研究表明，它参与感知了细胞内的氧含量。如果氧含量低，便会向周围细胞发送信号，开始生长新的血管。换句话说，它调节了血管的形成，这是肿瘤的一个重要特征（见图13）。进一步的研究表明，这些变化足以推动试管里的肿瘤细胞生长，而在这些模型中置换VHL基因就会逆转细胞的肿瘤特征。此外，在VHL综合征患者中发现的肾脏肿瘤类型叫肾细胞瘤，从该基因的功能便可预测，血管中显著富含肾细胞瘤。对散发（非遗传性）肾细胞瘤的研究表明，VHL基因在大约70%的病例中都突变了，这使得VHL基因/血管形成的路径成为诱人的治疗靶子。肾脏肿瘤一旦扩散就出名得难治，对基于VHL基因的新型疗法的研究则卓有成效：从2006年以来，有六种药物获得批准，还有好几种治疗某一疾病的药物正待获批；在过去的25年里，只有两种治疗此病的药物获得了许可。所有这些药物都把上文总结的遗传学研究所识别的路径当作攻击目标。

非遗传性癌症

尽管遗传性癌症为与癌症有关的基因类别提供了重要的线索，但大部分癌症病例却并非明显的遗传倾向所致。正如我们在第一章看到的那样，全世界癌症死亡的主要病因是肺、胃、肝、结肠以及乳腺的肿瘤。在这些癌症中，肺癌与吸烟密切相关，而肝癌则与乙型肝炎病毒感染有关，饮酒也扮演了重要角色。消化道癌症被认为与饮食有关，但明确的因果关系仍不甚了了。同样，乳腺癌（以及男性的前列腺癌）显然与饮食和激素因素有关。这些形形色色的影响是如何产生了上述变化，引发了癌症呢？

肺癌是环境中的致癌物相互作用而引发癌症的最好理解的例子。风险显然与吸烟量——存在着一种剂量效应——以及持续时间有关。吸烟者在患癌之前戒烟，戒断之后，患癌的风险会持续降低。根据福格尔斯泰因级联这样的模型，吸烟一定诱发了级联的第一阶段，而持续吸烟也必然会引发后续的阶段。在癌变的旧模型中，初始阶段往往被称为肿瘤生长的起始期，后续阶段被称为肿瘤生长的促进期，而最终阶段被称为癌化。这些术语仍有价值，在实验室里，使用药剂把非恶性的细胞生长变成肿瘤细胞的过程通常被称为细胞转化。对吸烟的分析表明，有很多药剂会在细胞培养系统中导致转化。对这些烟草成分的详细研究揭示了发生作用的精确分子机制，其精确程度直达与DNA双螺旋的相互作用模式。罪魁祸首之一被称为苯并芘，仔细研究表明，它会与DNA螺旋结合，破坏其结构。图15显示了与DNA双螺旋结合的苯并芘分子。

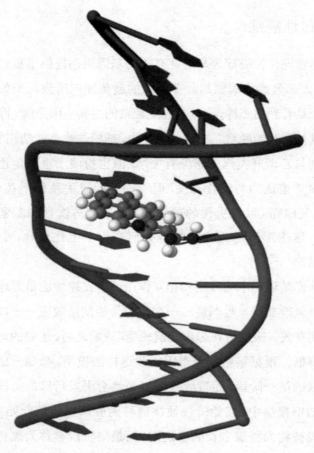

图15　与DNA结合的苯并芘

　　如上所述，在最终的癌变事件把癌前损伤变成成熟的肿瘤
40　之前，显然需要破坏DNA——这一初始事件之后，一般是进一
步破坏逐渐累积的延长期，有时被称为促进期。在烟草这个例
子中，这个过程似乎是由持续吸烟推动的，具有直接破坏DNA
的性质。对于其他疾病，特别是乳腺癌和前列腺癌，推动者的角

色是由个体自身的激素扮演的。正如第一章所指出的，乳腺癌的风险受到乳房受周期性雌激素刺激的时间的影响——因此，初潮较早、孕次较少且没有母乳喂养都会导致风险升高。由此推论，月经周期引发的乳房持续的周期性变化放大了某种形式的环境致癌物造成的任何对DNA的初始破坏。在前列腺癌中也可以看到类似的结果，与很可能接触了同样的环境致癌物的同龄人相比，幼年时期遭到阉割的男性（例如太监）患前列腺癌的风险非常低。酒精在肝癌中起到的作用也与之相似。如前所述，酒精不是直接的致癌物——它不会破坏DNA。然而，长期酗酒会诱发肝脏的损伤和修复周期，从而促进了细胞更新。就像乳房的周期性变化一样，这种不断增加的活动放大了必然存在的DNA损伤因子所造成的伤害，增加了DNA进一步累积损伤的机会，促成了癌症的发展。

如第一章所述，就肝癌而言，我们也已对最常见的致癌物——乙肝病毒感染——了如指掌。这种疾病在全世界都是一个巨大的痛苦来源，但在中国和亚洲其他地区尤甚，那里有高达10%的人口长期感染。印度和中东的感染率较低，而欧洲和北美的感染率则低于1%。长期感染的风险在那些婴儿时期便感染的人群中最高。自1982年起，乙肝疫苗已经问世。很多国家实施了多年的疫苗计划，才使科学家完成了一种病毒和癌症之间联系的最终试验——如果这种联系是因果性的，防止感染就应该也确实能预防这种疾病。病毒导致癌症的确切分子机制仍在研究之中，但就像吸烟一样，当前的因果证据足以令人信服。

接下来讨论另一种与感染有关的癌症——宫颈癌，可以看到相似的故事呼之欲出。1920年代人们发现，宫颈癌在性伴侣较多的女人中更常见，特别是妓女，而修女中则非常罕见（除了那些此前性事频繁的修女之外），这指向了一种性传播的感染性病因。1976年，哈拉尔德·楚尔·豪森证明，这种疾病与人乳头瘤病毒（HPV）感染有关。楚尔·豪森博士在生殖器疣和宫颈癌中均发现了HPV的DNA。他因为这一发现以及在该领域的后续工作而获得了诺贝尔医学奖，其研究显示了这种病毒和癌症之间确切的分子学联系。该病毒生成了与Rb和p53两个基因相互作用的各种蛋白质，这两个基因都是细胞周期的关键控制器，为肿瘤的产生提供了一条明显的路线。

针对HPV的疫苗研发（从而可预防宫颈癌），是比HBV疫苗更大的技术难题。然而，长期病毒感染和癌症之间的联系让宫颈癌癌前阶段的研究成为可能。人们发现，用木制刮片从子宫颈取得细胞涂片，随后在显微镜下检查，就可以对癌前阶段加以识别。名为宫颈上皮内瘤样病变（CIN）或原位癌（CIS）的癌前阶段识别促成了预防性的治疗。欧洲和北美大多数国家都有基于子宫颈涂片检查的全面筛检。据估计，这些计划拯救了数万人的生命。最近，一种针对与宫颈癌有关的各种HPV变体的疫苗在2006年面世，并作为防止感染的一个手段，开始出现在女孩的公共卫生疫苗计划之中，从而降低了癌症的风险。关于这种疫苗出现了一些争议，有人将其解读为防范性乱交风险的一个手段。然而，防范一种性传播疾病并不会降低人类感染免疫缺陷病毒（HIV）等其他疾病的风险。此外，该疫苗可以保护女人免于其伴侣此前的性乱交风险，毕竟她们对此毫无控制能力。但这种效果要等10到20年才能看到，因为这是HPV感染和癌症形成之间一贯的时间差。

癌症的治疗

　　癌症的治疗非常复杂，通常需要很多不同群体的参与，这些群体有各式各样的医生，包括全科医生（家庭医生）、外科医生、肿瘤学家、病理学家、放射科医生、临终关怀专家，以及大批其他专门人才——护士、放射师、理疗师、实验室和放疗科的技术人员、手术室护理员等等，不胜枚举。如何将这些不同群体具体组织起来，各国之间差别巨大，也是各国医疗卫生的政治和经济职能。

　　为了解决这个问题，我会把癌症治疗的组织呈现为一个历程，从症状出现到诊断、治疗、复查，最后还有对那些癌症复发不治之人的临终关怀。不同的医疗卫生系统处理这些事件的方式各不相同，但总的来说，基本原则是普遍适用的。本章的最后一部分概述了诸如外科手术、化疗和放疗等主要的治疗类别。45

初步诊断与调查

　　大多数患者主诉的仍然是诸如持续咳嗽等症状，或是尿血等问题。还有大量患者的问题是通过筛检计划查出的，要么是有组织有系统的筛检（例如乳腺癌和宫颈癌），要么是非正式的随机筛检（例如前列腺癌的PSA检查等）。有些病例是在调查其他问题时偶然发现的。例如，腹部扫描检查可能会发现肾脏的无症状肿瘤。后文中会再次讨论这些患者群体。

大多数患者会向医生描述他们自己注意到和担心的某种症状。虽然症状就像人一样五花八门，但通常可以分成两大类：一类是导致正常功能紊乱的异常症状，如会干扰正常行动的脑肿瘤；另一类是肿瘤造成损伤所导致的异常症状，如流血、疼痛或咳嗽。症状出现到确诊的时间可能非常短，有时也会达数年之久。诊断的延迟有时是因为卫生专业人士判断错误，有时是患者故意自我疏忽或自我欺骗，有时则是两者综合所致。

不出意料，错失早期诊断的时机，通常会在后来引发严重的医患关系问题，往往还是在最需要彼此配合的时候。在这方面，家庭医生就会遭遇很多麻烦。例如，头痛和背痛都是常见的症状，绝大多数病例的原因都是良性的，需要对症治疗而无须全面调查。当然，这些症状偶尔也会表明有潜在的脑部或脊柱肿瘤。另一个例子是便血。每一个医学生都知道这可能说明有肠癌。每一个家庭医生也都知道，对于处在"有一定风险"年龄段的患者来说，存在痔疮（刺激之下，肛门底部会出血）等状况实际上是非常普遍的。那么，他们如何在不对患者进行严重的过度检查的情况下，区分无关紧要的便血和严重（但罕见）的便血呢？答案往往在医学院传授的另一项基本功里——准确记录病史的技艺。因此，像混合在排便之中的严重出血这样突然而意外的变化就更可能归因于癌症，卫生纸上常年可见的少量鲜血涂迹则不然。

癌症筛检

在理想的世界里，我们能够提供检查，在癌症进入严重阶段之前识别出来，从而进行早期干预，治愈的希望也大得多。这种过程被称为筛检，如今可以针对乳腺癌、子宫癌、宫颈癌以及肠癌等多种癌症进行。此外，PSA血检为测试是否患上前列腺癌的筛检，但它的使用仍存在争议。描述一种理想筛检的特征，继而考察这些检测在实践中的发展过程，有助于我们深入了解它们。

下面的例子就说明了这一点：

表1　一种理想筛检的特征（来源：世界卫生组织）

- 目标疾病应是一种常见的癌症，相关死亡率很高
- 如果及早应用，应有能够降低死亡风险的有效治疗
- 检测程序应当易于接受、安全，并相对便宜

此外，我们需要考虑：

- 真阳性率：病人被正确诊断为患病
- 假阳性率：健康者被错误识别为患病
- 真阴性率：健康者被正确识别为健康
- 假阴性率：病人被错误识别为健康

表2　肝脏扫描结果和正确诊断之间的关系

	肝病患者	非肝病患者	合　计
肝脏扫描			
异常（＋）	231	32	263
正常（－）	27	54	81
合计	258	86	344

因此，灵敏性（有肝病且扫描异常的患者/扫描结果为阳性的全部患者）=231/（231+32）=0.88
而明确性（扫描正常且未患病的患者/扫描正常的全部患者）=54/（27+54）=0.67
另一个指标是阳性预测值（患有肝病的患者扫描异常的比例）=231/（231+27）=0.89
以及扫描结果为阴性的阴性预测值（未患肝病的患者扫描正常的比例）=54/（32+54）=0.63

对于临床测试来说，这个结果相当不错——疑似肝病患者的阳性扫描结果是此病患者的一个相当好的指标，表明此人患有肝病。那么，作为一种筛检，这样的结果如何呢？

为了说明使用一种检查来诊断已知患病之人与在无症状人群中筛检疾病之间的差异，可以观察一下乳腺癌的数字。假设接受检查人群的漏检率（特异度）是10%，而未检出的早期疾病水平是500人中有一人。如果我们现在检查100 000个人，理想的检查会在癌症患者中得到200个阳性检测结果，在未患此病的人群中得到99 800个阴性检测结果。然而我们的检查固然很好，却并不完美，在这200个病例中只会检出180个，让其余的20人错误地放了心。另一方面，该检查也并非完全特异。假设95%的未患病人群得到阴性的检测结果，但有5%的人会得到错误的阳性检测结果。当我们把这种情况应用到筛检人口中，就意味着在未患此病的99 800人中间，有5%的人得到了错误的阳性结果。可以计算得出，在未患此病的人群中有4 990个假阳性结果。这就是说，结果为阳性的人群中只有少数人（180/4 990 =4%）实际患有此病，而4 990−180 = 4 810个人都虚惊一场。此外，20个放错了心的人还会继续患有癌症，因为他们会认为自己没有患癌而忽视症状，可能在晚期才会检查出来。但是，取得阴性结果的绝大多数人（99 800人——超过99%）确实未患此病，因此，阴性的结果相当令人安心。

这些样例很重要，因为它们表明，筛检的局限性乍一看尚可接受。实际上，以上这些数字都是**最佳**的结果——灵敏度和特异度在年轻女性中双双下降（大概是因为她们的乳房组织更加密实，难以看清异常的肿块），导致错误分类的病例增多。此外，尽管检查本身所费无几，追踪假阳性的成本却要高得多，需要将其计入筛检计划的成本。

在考虑筛检的好处时，还有另一个问题。在上面的例子中，与没有筛检的情况相比，我们会较早地识别出一些癌症病例，这很可能使得治疗前景有所改善。然而，乳腺癌的治愈率相当好，四分之三的确诊女性都是长期存活者。这样一来，余下的四分之一注定不成功的患者成为筛检的主要潜在受益人。与参加检查的人数相比，这部分人数相对较少，而缺点则是未患乳腺癌的健康女性的过度检查问题。

对疑似癌症的调查

无论患者是经过筛检计划识别出来的，还是向医生陈述了令人担忧的症状，接下来都是进行进一步的检查，以确定或排除诊断结果。诊断通常基于受影响器官的组织样本（活检），此前则是由医生进行临床检查、成像以及血检。理想情况下，使用无创成像检查便可调查癌症。实际上，几乎所有病例的诊断都需要通过在实验室检查组织样本来确认。成像是决定在哪里以及如何获得组织的关键。要么使用X光——计算机断层成像（CT）扫描，要么使用核磁共振成像（MRI），得到的现代截面成像可以给出内部器官和疑似肿瘤的非常精细的图片。然而，就连最好的成像都不能确切地表明某个团块是否就是肿瘤，就算在极有可能得出癌症诊断的情况下，也不能确切表明癌症的种类。在偶然情况下，成像足以说明问题。例如，一位终身重度吸烟的瘦弱老者，X光胸片表示有疑似肺癌，而此人又不适合任何治疗，如此便可省去确诊活检的不适了。还有一两种情况也无

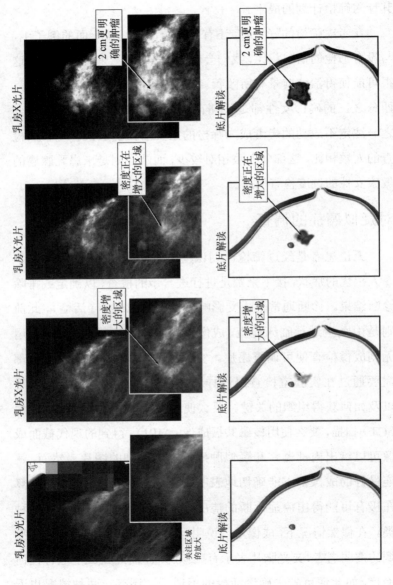

图 16 乳腺癌的乳房 X 光片

48

须活检——成像显示患者骨骼（前列腺癌扩散的常见位点）中有广泛的肿瘤沉积物，伴有血清前列腺特异抗原（PSA）水平大大升高，无须活检便能可靠地诊断为前列腺癌扩散。图例显示了乳房内的肿瘤标本扫描（图16）和肺脏与肝脏的继发性肿瘤病灶（图17）。在所有这些病例中，异常之处一目了然。但是，就算这些在放射学上明显的病变，一般也需要活检来确定癌症的具体类型，以及随后的恰当治疗。

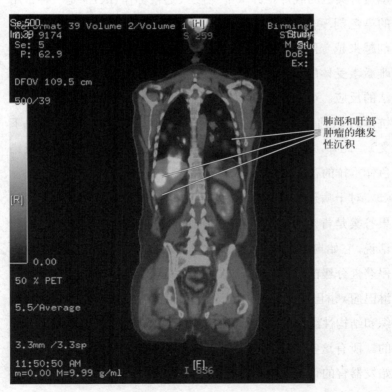

肺部和肝部肿瘤的继发性沉积

图17　患有晚期癌症并扩散到肺部和肝部的患者的CT/PET（正电子发射断层扫描）复合图像

病理科医生在癌症诊断中的作用

病理科医生评估的是少量的组织样本,比方说用采样针在活检中取得的样本。最初的材料偶尔可能来自手术切除的器官,例如在肾癌病例中,这种材料就可能来自患病的肾脏。通常是把移除肿瘤的非常薄的切片放在载片上,然后进行一系列染色,高亮显示引起关注的具体特点。随后,病理科医生便用显微镜检查染色的载片。苏木精-伊红(通常称作H&E)是一种常用的染色剂,可以高亮显示细胞核等细胞组分。如今使用的染色剂越来越专门化,这有助于进一步突出肿瘤的特点。乳腺癌中雌激素受体的染色就是一例,有助于预测肿瘤对化疗和激素疗法的反应。可用的检查数目迅速增加,大多数都是基于单克隆抗体的(它们作为治疗的形式,其数量也在迅速增加——参见下文)。此外,为了寻找特定基因表达的变化,或是特定突变或染色体重排的存在,也都可以进行检查。

对于病理科医生而言,主要的问题是:"这是肿瘤吗?"如果答案是肯定的,那么接下来的问题包括具体的类型——换句话说,它始自哪个器官,以及它是什么亚型。此外,肿瘤是根据侵袭性分级的,通常从一级(低)到三级(高)。例如前列腺癌、淋巴瘤(淋巴腺的癌症),以及肉瘤(骨骼、肌肉或软骨等结缔组织和结构性组织的癌症)等癌症的分级系统不同,但原理是一样的。所有这些系统都基于肿瘤细胞的规模和形状,以及它们与始发器官的正常细胞相比有何差异。

近来越来越多的附加次级分类以肿瘤出现的分子标记物为基础。根据在肿瘤本身或血液循环(有时在尿液中也会出现)

癌
症

中特定标记的超标水平，它们可以被定义为标志性特征。分子标记物最广为人知的例子大概就是乳腺癌中的HER2了。1980年代末，洛杉矶加州大学的丹尼斯·斯莱门博士首次将其描述为乳腺癌和卵巢癌预后不佳的一个标记。这促成了药物曲妥珠单抗（赫赛汀）的研发，针对的就是这种蛋白质含量过高的细胞（术语称之为过度表达）。起初在患有晚期疾病的患者中间，后来又在新近确诊的患者中间进行的里程碑式的试验表明，该药物显著改善了25%的HER2蛋白质含量高的患癌女性的结果。因此，对HER2表达的肿瘤样本染色就能提供重要的预后信息，同时也有助于指导对治疗的选择。

病理科医生在癌症治疗中的另一个重要作用，是对来自手术切除的患癌器官的样本进行评估。上文提出的问题会以更大的样本重新评估，除此之外，病理科医生还要解决下列问题：

- 肿瘤是否仅限于手术切除的器官？
- 手术的切缘（样本的边缘）是否没有肿瘤的存在？
- 是否扩散到关联结构，如淋巴腺？

治疗决策

完成活检和适当的成像之后，必须要对患者的治疗手段做出决策了。重要的初步决定是治愈是否可行。如果治疗基本上是为了减轻病痛，这必须在决策时加以考虑——生活质量就成为首要的目标。如果治疗有可能治愈，那么就要另外考虑了——研究表明，患者为了治愈付出的代价可能是忍受相当大的副作用。无论目标是治愈、延长生命，或是缓解症状，都有一系列手段可供使用，既可单独使用，也可以组合进行。决策需要定期复核，治疗也需根据副作用和肿瘤反应——也就是说，情况是否改善——来进行调整。

在各大卫生系统中，这些决策越来越不是由医生个人做出的，而是由通常缩写为MDT的多学科团队进行的（在当今的英国，如果医院要报销癌症治疗费用，就必须如此）。一般来说，这些团队会由外科医生、放射和肿瘤内科医生、放射科医生、病理科医生，以及专科护士组成。在与患者商讨评价各种检查结果之前，MDT会先行复核基准信息（术语称之为阶段信息）。大体而言，这些决策会根据国家或国际的最佳实践准则而定。然后会在诊所与患者讨论结果和治疗选择，最终确定临床方案。

我们会依次介绍不同的治疗模式，但在开始之前，对治疗模式的相对重要性做一个大概的分类，或许会有所裨益。图18预测了100位"普通"患者在现代西方医疗系统中的治疗模式。显然，这些数字只是供说明之用，各国情况不同，甚至在有着地方惯例的同一个国家里也不尽相同。例如，治疗膀胱癌既可以通过外科手术摘除膀胱（膀胱切除术），也可通过放疗破坏肿瘤，外科手术可以作为放疗失败的后备补救方案。在美国，很少有患者在可选的情况下接受放疗，后者通常是保留给老弱病患做缓解治疗的（控制症状）。相反，在英国，大约有三分之二的患者主要接受放疗，而手术主要针对更合适的年轻患者。这种主流做法上的差异主要源自英美卫生业的差别（参见第五章），而不是任何基于证据的差别。

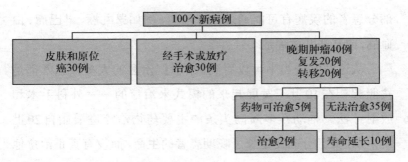

图18 癌症治疗在不同治疗模式上的分布

分布比例背后的基本原则是，大约30%的病例只是非常局部的侵袭——如基底皮肤癌（通常称作侵蚀性溃疡）——只需要非常有限的局部治疗，一般采用手术，但偶尔也会采取放疗。在余下的病例中，大约有40%的患者的肿瘤会广泛扩散，还有30%患有局部晚期肿瘤，可以通过手术或放疗等局部/区域性治疗予以根除。如前所示，精确的分布比例各不相同，部分是地理原因，但也因解剖部位的变化而不同。例如，手术是治疗肠癌的最佳手段，而不是放疗，因为正常的大肠对放疗的耐受度相对较差，何况以活动结构为靶向显然问题重重。另一方面，如今宫颈癌的主要治疗手段是放疗结合同步进行的化疗，并把手术作为后备的补救方案。另外，评估该病是否造成了局部扩散也起到了有限的作用。

在癌症发展进入晚期的患者中，大约有半数从一开始便体现出这一点，另外半数开始时患有明显的局部疾病，但随后旧病复发，问题广泛扩散。在晚期（一般称为转移性）的癌症患者中，大多数人患上的基本上都是不治之症。这些疾病像晚期的肺癌、肠癌、乳腺癌、前列腺癌或肝癌，都是主要的癌症杀手。少部分患者的疾病有可能通过化疗治愈,例如睾丸癌、淋巴瘤、白血病,或某些儿童癌症。

从这样的分类中可以看到,21世纪治愈的大多数患者都是按照起初在19世纪发展起来的模式来治疗的——外科手术和放射疗法。推动众多新闻头条的主要药物治疗进展始自20世纪中期,大部分药物延长了晚期患者的生命,而没有真正治愈他们。公共卫生领域的医生们熟知这一事实,大众却对此不甚满意。由此可知,在比较贫困的国家,只有实施良好的基础外科手术和放疗才会取得对癌症的最大影响。直肠癌在全世界的存活率就最好地证明了这一点。古巴治疗该病取得的结果最佳,众所周知,该国的医疗护理组织相当完善,但它获得更加昂贵的新药的途径却非常有限。在资源有限的地区,癌症化疗最好集中关注儿童白血病和睾丸癌等罕见的化疗可治愈的癌症。因为这些癌症主要发生于年轻人群,在这一领域的药物支出对于所拯救的生命年限的影响要高得多,远非拯救老年患者的临终癌症药物支出可比。老年人的晚期疾病药物疗法,对治愈率的影响往往要小得多。就算治愈属寻常之事,患者本身已届老龄,无论怎样,其预期寿命都更加有限。第五章将会详细讨论这个主题。

外科手术

外科手术显然有上千年的历史了,但癌症手术的时代实际上可以追溯到19世纪中期有效麻醉的出现,外科手术由此从孤注一掷、"鲜血淋漓"的可怕的紧急截肢,发展成为可受控制的解剖。如上所述,移除肿瘤的手术是癌症治疗的支柱之一(此外还有放疗），尽管药物治疗已有进步，在可预见的未来，情况似乎仍然如此。外科医生在日益发展微创（常被称为锁眼）手术技术，无需大切口便可进行。这些手术的优势是术后恢复迅速，但的确增加了手术次数，技术难度也增加了。因为恢复时间较短，这些技术使得老弱患者可以接受手术。还因为恢复期的痛苦较

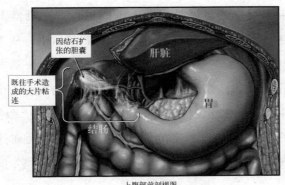

因结石扩张的胆囊

既往手术造成的大片粘连

肝脏

胃

结肠

上腹部前剖视图

开腹胆囊切除术
以粘连松解术打开切口，切除胆囊

腹腔镜胆囊切除术
因为过度粘连而未执行

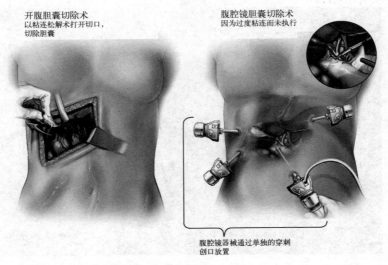

腹腔镜器械通过单独的穿刺创口放置

图 19　开放式与腹腔镜胆囊切除术的对比

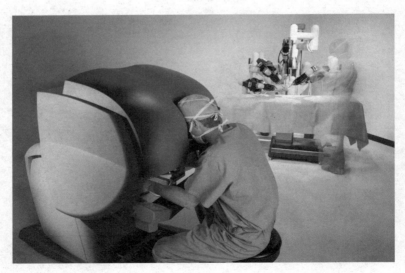 少以及完全恢复正常功能的康复期较短，它们对所有患者群体都更具吸引力。与此相反，用金属长管进行手术，并用一种改良的望远镜进行窥视被比喻为用筷子系鞋带，这使得开刀手术的

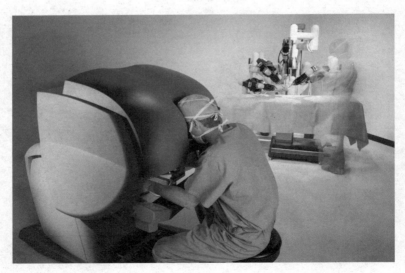58 支持者声称，关键的癌症治疗效果可能会打折扣——例如肿瘤的完整移除。对这方面治疗的评估由病理科医生完成——那可是癌症团队的关键成员。

微创手术近来的进展是机器人辅助过程。在机器人手术中，手术器械是人工插入的，随后便固定在机器臂上。插入观察孔后，外科医生就在与患者隔离的控制台上操作——基本上是使用计算机游戏技术来远程操纵器械。这种激动人心的技术也有潜在的缺点，例如，机器人器械的设置比直接操纵"微创"器械耗时还长。另外，机器本身要价100万英镑左右，每年还需大约15万英镑的运营费用。这是一笔相当大的额外开支，远远超

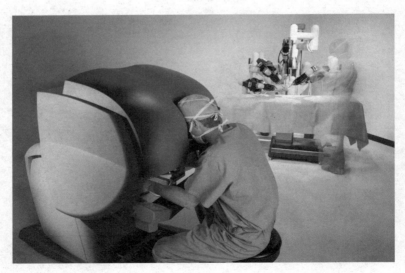

图20　机器人辅助的外科手术

出了手术室、病房、麻醉科等部门的一般基础设施的全部费用。这种技术最终是否既能取得临床效果，又具备成本效益，显然还有待观察。当然，美国如今对机器人手术有着非常强烈的消费者/患者需求，或许最终能战胜冷酷的临床考虑。59

放射疗法

放射疗法是19世纪的另一项技术，其势头在21世纪依然强劲。1895年，伦琴的重要观察为现代放射疗法奠定了基础。他发现，当朝着真空里的一个目标发射电子时，产生了不可见的光线（他称之为"X光"）——这些光线能让感光胶片变黑。人们很快意识到，X光传递了能量，而这种能量有望用于治疗和成像。短短数月后，第一批皮肤肿瘤患者就得到了治疗，创新的速度惊心动魄。成像和治疗的技术在过去一个多世纪里逐渐完善提高，如今已经是现代癌症疗法的关键组成部分。的确，如前所述，现代癌症疗法最有效的部分仍是外科手术和放射疗法，外加在治愈率方面相对次要的药物治疗。在富裕的第一世界国家，药物治疗得到的资金支持显然远超这两种关键的核心疗法。然而，比较贫穷的国家不得不做出艰难的选择，与外科手术和放射疗法相比，鲜有药物可以在治疗方面提供出色的性价比。

在对电生成或使用放射性同位素产生的X光效果进行初步观察之后，这种技术逐步得到了完善。起初的技术是基于伦琴在19世纪描述的真空管，它能发射穿透到内脏的光束，但在皮肤附近沉积了极大剂量。1950年代，更加强大的所谓兆伏机面世了。这些机器使用的是人工同位素钴-60，现在已被所谓直线加

速器（一般简写为linac）这种电气设备所取代。后一种机器使
用了二战时为雷达研发的磁控阀。脉冲可以以高得多的能量把
电子"轰"进靶位，治疗深部肿瘤的性能好得多——仿佛是高科
技刀剑上的电子犁刃。

通过用细部成像来整合治疗的实施，现代放疗可以做到非
常精确的定位。副作用有两方面。在皮肤、消化道内膜和口腔
等结构，效果可比晒伤，严重程度取决于吸收的剂量。感受的效
果取决于治疗的部位，可能会包括低位肠道治疗引发的腹泻，或
口疮、脱发，以及接受治疗的皮肤部位变红等等。第二组副作用
体现在肺脏和肾脏等实体结构上。对这些器官的治疗几乎没有
即时的效果，但如果超过了临界剂量限制，被照射的组织会逐渐
失能。因此，靶位肿瘤附近的重要器官接受的剂量就成了放疗
实施的关键限制——为了治疗癌症，一定量的毒性是值得接受
的，但显然存在一个破坏大于收益的临界点。调强放疗（IMRT）
等改善的放疗专注于非常复杂的计量配比，看起来在重要的结
构周围"改变"了剂量，其应用越来越普遍，但实施的成本和复
杂度也随之上升。一项有关的发展是治疗机器的板载成像，它
可以被用来实施图像引导放疗（IGRT），其中治疗能够每天跟踪
肿瘤的移动。IMRT与IGRT的组合有望既能（通过确保治疗射
中靶位）提高对肿瘤的控制，又能更好地绕过不相关的组织，从
而降低副作用。

激素疗法

尽管如今化疗在癌症药物疗法中占据主导地位，但首个成
功的癌症治疗药物却是一种基于激素的药物疗法。癌症的激素

疗法可以追溯到1940年代，来自美国泌尿科医生查尔斯·哈金斯在晚期前列腺癌患者身上的发现。

　　激素疗法的先驱们推断，如果"母本"组织需要正常的激素水平，那么来自组织的异常肿瘤或许也保留了这种依赖性。在晚期前列腺癌患者身上所做的去势试验产生了惊人的结果，骨骼中的癌症病灶所引起的疼痛等症状得到了迅速而显著的改善。此后，医生尝试使用了当然会抑制雄性特征的雌激素，再次获得了惊人结果。可惜的是，这些激素的效果尽管显著，却只能维持一两年，随后疾病就会复发。患有乳腺癌的绝经期前女性，在切除卵巢后也观察到了类似的结果。后来的几十年里，出现了各种具体针对前列腺癌和乳腺癌的基于激素的药物疗法。其中一种药物，即雌激素阻滞剂他莫昔芬，挽救的生命大概比其他任何抗癌药物都多。半个多世纪过去了，针对激素路径的新药仍在临床上不断出现。

化学疗法

　　如果请大众说出与癌症治疗关系最密切的药物种类，他们一定会说是化疗。这个术语涵盖大量不同的药剂，来源十分广泛，从抗生素到植物提取物，再到基于DNA人工合成的化学制剂。所有这些药物都会干预细胞分裂的机制，并且由于很多组织都有正在分裂的细胞，因而会导致恶心与呕吐（一部分原因是消化道内膜遭到破坏，另一部分原因是大脑受到了直接影响）、脱发（对毛囊的破坏）等典型的副作用，以及感染的风险（抵御感染所需的白细胞的产生遭到了破坏）。我们都十分熟悉（用 62 通俗小报的说法是）与癌症"作战"的光头患者的形象。虽说化疗中的确会发生这种情形,实际情况却更加多样,在门诊条件下实施的很多化疗几乎不会造成恶心或脱发。脱发很难预防,但它并非所有化疗药物的统一特性。如今,恶心与呕吐在很大程度上都可以预防,这样患者就可以服用迄今被认为毒性过大的药物,就连上了年纪的患者也一样。这非常重要,因为很多化疗都是为了缓解症状,因而生活质量是重中之重。如果生活质量很差,延长生命就没有什么意义了。

第一批化疗药物是基于从芥子气中取得的化学物质研制的,芥子气曾在第一次世界大战期间被广泛使用,效果相当恐怖。据说,接触过这些药剂的士兵生还后会出现白细胞(血液中负责抵御感染的细胞)数量下降的情况。当然也有人患上了一种白细胞的癌症,也就是通常所谓的白血病。人们用氮芥等芥子气衍生物,在白血病和一种叫作淋巴瘤的次级相关组的癌症上进行了很多试验。这些试验中的患者第一次体验到一些状况减轻了,这些状况在此前根本无法治疗。不幸的是,在单独用药的情况下,状况的缓解只是暂时的。但试验证明,进一步用药之后,这些药物组合使用最终可能会治愈白血病和淋巴瘤患者。

随后出现了一波新的化疗药物,在1970年代和1980年代,人们普遍认为这些药物会继而促成针对大多数晚期癌症的治愈疗法。这些药物的来源多种多样。植物提取物(长春新碱、多西他赛、紫杉醇)、络合重金属(顺铂、卡铂),以及抗生素(阿霉素、丝裂霉素)等被证明是卓有成效的探索领域,带来了多个大规模实验室筛检计划,在大量的植物和细菌提取物中寻找有希望的化学药物。另一个探索领域是从DNA或细胞分裂过程的其他

63

构件中取得的化合物,最佳的例子就是RNA的组分之一(见第二章)、尿嘧啶的衍生物——5-氟尿嘧啶(5FU)。分子中额外的氟原子让5FU得以与DNA和RNA发生作用,却无法被正常加工——在此过程中相当于一个分子"扳手"。

　　1970年代和1980年代取得了进一步的显著成功,特别是晚期睾丸癌,从一种致命疾病变成了一种高治愈率的病症。如此巨大成功的最好说明,就是环法自行车赛冠军七度获得者兰斯·阿姆斯特朗,他被确诊患上了广泛扩散的疾病,连大脑也被侵袭了。大量化疗取得成功后,他继续参赛,赢得了他的第一个环法赛冠军,其后又是打破纪录的六次夺冠。各种白血病和很多儿童癌症上也见证了类似的成功。然而不幸的是,主要的癌症杀手更耐化疗,虽说大多数肿瘤类型都会在一定程度上对化疗有所反应,这些癌症却难以治愈。有人认为,问题或许在于化疗的药物没有给到足够的剂量。但是,1990年代的一轮试验表明,就算极大剂量的化疗药物组合加上骨髓移植,也无法治愈晚期乳腺癌等主要杀手。

　　这一认识引发了研究重点的变化。晚期疾病尽管无法治愈,却会在一段时间内对化疗作出反应,这一观察促使人们在早期疾病的环境下测试化学疗法,就像以前在激素疗法中的做法一样。我们知道,很多无明显疾病的患者后来却出现了复发。这表明一定有非常少量的肿瘤潜伏下来未被发现。研究者假定,在早期实施化疗可能比等检测到复发再做化疗的效果 64 要好。初步试验的结果令人失望,但事后发现,这只是因为成效过小,难以察觉。当乳腺癌的试验结果汇集起来,人们认识到早期化疗是有效的,与把化疗作为"补救"治疗的人相比,接受早期化疗的女性复发间隔和存活时间都较长。这叫作辅助疗法，其根据是所谓的"微转移"疾病可以根除的原理，而一旦扫描可见，疾病便无法治愈了。现代的扫描仪器尽管非常灵敏，却基本上无法检测出直径小于数毫米的肿瘤。因此，我们无法区分哪些是首次手术或化疗便已治愈的人，哪些是扫描显示正常，但实际上藏有少量残留的肿瘤病灶、未来注定会导致复发的人。后续研究改进了使用的药物组合，也改善了获益最多的女性群体的状况。辅助疗法的问题在于，很多女性只接受外科手术和放疗就已取得了不错的效果，因而化疗对她们没有任何好处，只有毒性和潜在的伤害。这种风险对疾病复发风险最低的人是最高的，无论复发风险低是源于疾病的侵袭性较低，还是源于死于其他原因的风险较高（例如非常年迈的人）。

近来，人们更加重视化疗对于症状缓解所起的作用。这看似矛盾——施用有毒的药物来减少痛苦。然而，症状控制的改善，特别是使用药物防止此前与化疗相伴的严重恶心，改变了这些缓解药物的价值。生存时限的提高往往相对适度——通常只有数月，这使得研究人员研发了衡量生命质量的方法。如此，就能在产生益处（例如减轻痛苦）的有毒药物和常常被总称为"最佳支持治疗"的替代药物（止痛药、放疗，诸如此类）之间进行比较了。

辅助和缓解这两个使用趋势，大大增加了发达世界的癌症药物费用（见第五章），尽管收益相对较小，获益之人的数目却极为可观，因此如今相对年长的癌症患者也开始广泛使用化疗了。

单克隆抗体

抗体是动物体免疫防御的关键组成部分。每个抗体都由一个恒定区和一个可变区组成。可变区负责把抗体与其目标结合起来，如图21所示。抗体的正常功能是与入侵的感染有机体（病毒、细菌等）结合。接触到新的感染有机体后，机体的白细胞将其识别出来，并选择最能粘住入侵者并令其失能的具有抗体可变区的细胞（称作淋巴细胞）。相关细胞的生产大幅增加，随之增加了能够与入侵者结合的抗体的产量。一旦结合，其他的免疫细胞就将抗体的恒定区作为把它们拉出体循环的"钩子"，识别出抗体包覆的入侵者并吞噬它们。免疫系统的进化是复杂多细胞有机体生存所必需的关键演化步骤之一。免疫系统天生有缺陷的人很难在儿童时期存活下来，彰显了这个功能的重要性。

1970年代，技术得到了发展，可以通过制造与肿瘤细胞等"人造"目标相拮抗的抗体来利用免疫系统的能力。这些人工设计的靶向抗体被称作单克隆抗体——由单一的细胞克隆而来的抗体——可以粘在几乎任何被选中的靶位上。通过选择肿瘤细胞上的靶位，这些天然的分子既可通过连接放射性化学物质来帮助成像，又可直接凭借自身能力进行治疗。

当单克隆抗体首次面世时，人们以为它将成为"灵丹妙药"，可以为每一种肿瘤量身定制，从而根除晚期癌症。很遗憾，事实没有那么戏剧化，不过30年后，如今有越来越多的单克隆抗体投入了临床应用。

最广为人知的单克隆抗体大概就是曲妥珠单抗了，它更常用的名字是商品名赫赛汀。这种药物以肿瘤细胞表面上一种名

66

67

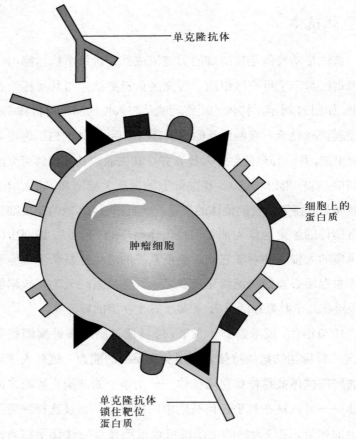

单克隆抗体

细胞上的
蛋白质

肿瘤细胞

癌
症

单克隆抗体
锁住靶位
蛋白质

图21 附着在肿瘤细胞上的单克隆抗体简图

为HER2的蛋白质为攻击对象，后者是被称为生长因子受体的一族蛋白质的成员。最好将它们想象成由循环蛋白（在本例中称作调蛋白）所调节的开关。大约有三分之一的乳腺肿瘤细胞表面有一种形式异常的HER2，基本上会导致开关被永久地"打开"了。HER2呈阳性的乳房肿瘤比HER2阴性的肿瘤生长得更快，也更具侵袭性。因此，以细胞表面的HER2为靶子似乎是个合乎逻辑的策略，而单克隆抗体则是实现该策略的妙法。起初的研究在患有HER2阳性肿瘤的女性中进行，并确认行之有效，该药物在2002年获得了批准。结果虽然是好的，可以观察到肿瘤缩小了，却不像期待的那样激动人心。尽管如此，人们认为进一步的试验值得一试，这一次将赫赛汀与化疗联合用于治疗晚期疾病。这些试验产生了更加惊人的结果，与那些只接受化疗的人相比，接受赫赛汀治疗的女性存活时间延长了大约50%。

下一阶段的研发结果更有趣。在证明了对不治之症的益处之后，下一个步骤就是在处于有望治愈阶段的早期患者中测试该药物，这种策略在激素疗法和化疗中已经取得了成功。赫赛汀辅助试验取得了肿瘤学上的成功，复发风险减半，某些此前无法治愈的女性也出现了被真正治愈的可能。但其中暗藏陷阱。患有HER2阳性的早期乳腺癌的大多数女性实际上只需接受手术、放疗和化疗，前景便已一片光明。如果一位女性已经通过这些治疗而痊愈了，她显然不会从任何进一步的治疗中获益（实际上还有可能受到伤害，因为赫赛汀带有导致心脏病的风险）。

反过来，即便接受了当前所有的疗法，有些女性仍会死亡，因此她们的获益也相对很少。处于两者之间的才是真正的赢家：原本注定会旧病复发，现在却有可能痊愈。这意味着在辅助（预防性）的环境中，需要很多人接受治疗，才能使一个真正的赢家受益，比例可能会高达20∶1。因为赫赛汀的价格很高（每年大约30 000英镑），每拯救一位女性的有效成本预计便达20×30 000 = 600 000英镑左右。因此当这种药物获批用于辅助治疗时，新一轮激烈的争论随之而来，也就不足为奇了——为了挽救一个生命,花费多少钱才是合理的?

靶向分子疗法

DNA革命和整个人类基因组的测序一直承诺其裨益会带来更好的药物。随着越来越多的基因被克隆,为异于正常细胞的肿瘤细胞基因绘制图谱指日可待。一旦识别了某个关键基因,随后便可设计出药物以这种异常基因为目标,或者更准确地说,以其关联的蛋白质产物为靶子。如上所述,靶向疗法的一种方式是使用抗体。另一种方式如今促成了大量新药问世,那就是制造干预功能的化学物质,无论干预的是异常蛋白质本身的功能,还是细胞中同一路径上某个其他部分的功能。前一种策略的第一个或许也是最好的例子,就是白血病药物伊马替尼(格列卫)。长期以来人们一直认为,一种名为慢性淋巴细胞白血病(CLL)的疾病的特征是存在所谓的"费城染色体"。这种异常的染色体来自两个不同染色体的融合,结果就产生了一种来自两种不同基因的异常蛋白质——bcr-abl融合蛋白质。详细的分子生物学研究证明,bcr-abl是驱动CLL细胞的必要和充分条件(这是研发候选新药的关键条件),使其成为理想的靶子。伊马替尼是成功命中目标的第一种药物,它改变了CLL的预后,那些已经对前期使用的化疗药物产生耐药性的患者的缓解期延长了。但不幸的是,尽管缓解期有所延长,却并非永久性的——肿瘤细胞最终还是会耐药。这是靶向小分子疗法的一个特点——它们往往非常有效,与化疗相比副作用较低,但一般不会治愈。然而,如我们在化学疗法一节中谈到白血病时提到的,初次单独使用这些药物也只会缓解而非治愈,所以希望组合使用能够证

69

明同样是有利的。时间会证明一切。

靶向疗法的第二种做法是瞄准与"核心"异常有关联的路径。这种做法的最佳范例是肾癌疗法近来的转变。直到最近，晚期肾癌几乎还是无法治愈，只有干扰素和白细胞介素-2这两种药物获批上市，药效都非常有限。大多数肾癌的发生都是"自发性"的，也就是说，家族其他成员不会患上同一种癌症。人们在多年前就已经观察到，家族成员长出相同肿瘤是非常罕见的，往往在幼年就发生了——见第二章关于遗传性癌症的章节。冯希佩尔和林道描述过这样一种遗传性综合征，该综合征如今就以他们的名字命名。作为疾病的一部分，冯希佩尔-林道（VHL）综合征患者会发展出多种早期肾癌。在微观层面上，VHL的各种癌症与更加常见的非遗传性癌症很相似，因此，人们怀疑VHL基因的异常情况或许在自发性癌症中也存在，事实证明的确如此。然而，VHL综合征患者的问题在于VHL蛋白质的正常功能**缺失了**；因此，以VHL蛋白质本身为靶子只会让问题变得更糟。对VHL路径的研究表明，VHL功能低下的一个结果是，通常受到VHL蛋白质抑制的各种蛋白质变得过度活跃了。其中包括驱动细胞分裂的蛋白质，以及另一族推动新血管产生的分子。以这条路径上失灵的VHL蛋白质的上游或下游成员为目标的药物被研发出来，其中包括三种小分子疗法，即舒尼替尼、索拉非尼和替西罗莫司，以及一种名为贝伐珠单抗的单克隆抗体。

70

这些药物的试验引发了晚期肾癌治疗的革命，自2006年以来，四种药物均获得了批准，还有一系列新的药物正在走向临床。然而，就像CLL一样，虽然大的晚期肿瘤首次缩小了，但这些药物在大多数病例中并不能治愈，耐药性也会随时间而不断升高。如今的试验重点关注辅助疗法、测序和组合施药，希望能够实现更大的存活收益。

　　与上文赫赛汀的故事一样，这些药物高昂的成本引起了巨大的争议——患者需要持续治疗而不是被施以有限的疗程，如同以前化疗等疗法的常规做法。药物非常昂贵——每年的治疗需要25 000到30 000英镑——获取药物的手段也会随之发生变化（见第五章）。然而，与赫赛汀和乳腺癌不同，加拿大、澳大利亚、苏格兰和英格兰等国的采购当局对呼声不断的女性乳腺癌游说的反应相当积极，却对资助一群以老年男性患者为主的群体接受治疗较为抵触。

用于控制症状的药物

　　在过去的10到15年里，一系列支持性治疗药物尽管不能直接治疗癌症，却也促成了癌症治疗的巨大进步。上文已经提到过得到改善的抗恶心药物。同样与化疗的安全性和实施有关的是生长因子，特别是可以提高白细胞数量、降低感染风险的粒细胞集落刺激因子（G–CSF）。第二个有关的产物名为GM–CSF（粒细胞–巨噬细胞集落刺激因子），起初是为同样的目的而研发的，后来却证明在把名为干细胞的血细胞前体释放到循环系统中起到了很有价值的作用。这种有些深奥难解的观察，使得专业人员可以在实施旨在破坏正常骨髓的高剂量化疗之前，先行采集干细胞。此前患者需要进行骨髓移植以在接受此种治疗前"拯救"他们，但结果证明，采集到的干细胞也能达到同样的效果，速度却更快，治疗前的采集过程也要容易得多，从而扩大了适合接受这些高剂量疗法的患者群。

71

近来研究的另一个领域是骨保护剂。很多扩散到骨骼的肿瘤都有着毁灭性的后果,包括疼痛、骨折,以及脊柱损伤所致的瘫痪。研究表明,一个悖论是,身体对肿瘤的"过度反应"会导致损伤增加。起初为骨质疏松症研发的药物结果却可以减少这种附加的自残性损伤。最初可用的药物如氯膦酸盐的效价相对较低,但后来的唑来膦酸和伊班膦酸等药物,其效价要高很多倍,可以大幅降低晚期肿瘤患者的骨损伤。更有趣的是,在高风险乳腺癌的辅助试验中,唑来膦酸似乎也减少了软组织疾病,表明这些药剂或许还有直接的抗癌性质。

结 语

100年来,癌症治疗取得了巨大进步,改变了全世界数百万人的治疗结果。与50年前或100年前相比,21世纪初的癌症治疗更加安全、高效,毒性也更低。手术和放疗仍在不断改进和提高,更好的靶向和微创技术也越来越多。辅助成像和病理学服务也会继续改善,未来会有更好的治疗选择。药物的种类及其有效性正在迅速增加,这将会在未来数年里带来更大的进步。就像我们要在第五章讨论的那样,所有这些进展的主要问题在于成本的飙升,但应对这个问题总好过毫无选择。

72

癌症研究

引　言

　　正如我们已经看到的那样，癌症疗法的支柱仍是手术和放疗，两者都可以追溯到19世纪，但也都经历了持续的技术改进过程，而且目前仍在进步。相较而言，癌症的药物治疗则是更加晚近的事。第一个成功的癌症药物疗法是在1940年代使用人工合成的雌激素来治疗前列腺癌。成功的治愈性化疗实际上可以追溯到1970年代，当时研发了针对白血病和淋巴瘤（骨髓和淋巴系统的肿瘤）的治疗方法，然而有趣的是，这些方法所使用的化学药物此前却是为了不道德的目的而研发的（正如我们看到的，该领域首批成功的药物之一氮芥就来自芥子气的活性成分）。新治疗手段的研发和现有治疗手段的改善显然需要研究的过程。本章将会描述某些研发的方式，特别是药物的规则与设备（如放疗仪器）或技术（外科手术）的规则之间的差异。我们将详细探讨这些差异，因为有些重要的差别会产生显著的异

常。本章将重点关注新的治疗手段从何而来，但类似的试验结
构适用于现有治疗手段之间的相互检验，也适用于对症状控制
技术的研究。

新的手术和放疗技术的研发过程与药物的研发过程大不相
同。一般来说，手术的改进将是技术上的一个小变化（例如，控
制出血的更佳方法），不会从根本概念上改变基础的技术。这样
的改进能否获批的根据往往是"目的适用性"（也就是说，它是
否真的有助于控制出血？）。同样的理由也适用于技术性放疗
的改进（例如，靶向放射而不损害正常组织的更佳做法）。总体
而言，这些类型的改进必须更好，随后也会付诸实践，这被认为
是不言而喻的。实际上，这些改进也许只是错觉，推进其实施的
可能是商业压力，而非任何合理的证据基础。我会用机器人手
术技术和调强放疗为例，说明这种情况发生的起源和原因。

另一方面，药物治疗则必须满足全然不同的标准。一般来
说，美国的食品药品监督管理局（FDA）这样的监管机构要求，
存活率与以前的治疗标准相比必须要有一定的提高。这意味着
一种新的药物治疗需要进行一系列临床试验的检测，有大量患
者参与其中。这些试验大体上可以分成三个类别，称为一期到
三期。

一期试验证明一种药物的安全性和副作用属性。一般来
说，只有少数患者参与该期试验，就癌症药物而言，他们通常都
是那些已经尝试尽了标准选项以及此前已接受过多种治疗方法
的人。副作用不太严重的药物，如降血压药，往往会先在健康的
志愿者身上进行测试。二期试验规模更大，与一期研究的参与
者相比，这一期参与者的"癌症之旅"往往还在较早期，试验的目

第四章 癌症研究

的在于确认一种药物对目标癌症具备有用的活性。对于看起来很有希望的药物来说，最终的三期试验会将其与被认定为治疗标准的任何项目进行比较。一次三期试验会有数百乃至数千患者参与。这样的设计本身就有很多问题，从批准文件、成本到法律负担等等。三期的批准试验如今几乎都是国际事务，必须遵守多个国家的法律框架，特别是美国的。这种试验成本巨大，也就解释了新药的昂贵——一种癌症新药从合成到注册要花费大约10亿美元。批准的过程——给予公司在市场上营销一种药物或产品，并从中获利的权利——受到FDA等国家或跨国机构的严格监管。下一章将会进一步讨论监管这个主题，可以说，对试验的高水平监管保护了试验的个体参与者免受可能的伤害，却让整个社会付出了代价，即拖慢了改进的步伐，并把新药的成本抬高到获取日益受限的地步，就算在最富裕的国家也是如此。

研发癌症新药

基础科学

显然，癌症研究有着体量庞大的生物研究的支持。过去50年里生物研究取得了巨大的进步，特别是DNA结构和所谓的生物学"中心法则"的解读，即第二章详细讨论过的DNA、RNA和蛋白质的关系。前几代癌症药物基本上都是通过观察化学物质对细胞的影响来进行研发的，目的是寻求对杀死肿瘤细胞特别有效的药物。这种研究产生了1970年代和1980年代大量出现的化疗药物。虽说新的化疗药剂现在仍在生产，但与前几十年取得的巨大进步相比，近来的药物给人以回报减少的感觉。

近来的研究重点，是与目标小分子和单克隆抗体有关的肿瘤分子标签的最新知识,上一章讨论过相关内容。20世纪末,人们对人类基因组进行了测序。最初的测序技术笨拙而缓慢,第一个完整的序列花了很多年才完成。这项任务完成之后,如今在了解了人类基因组整体结构的情况下,就有可能给具体癌症的基因组测序,并将癌变DNA和提取自患者血细胞的正常DNA进行比较了。如今,专门的实验室团队只需短短几周就能完成这一任务,成本也在迅速下降。在接下来的几年里,技术、所需时间以及成本都很可能取得惊人的改进,以至于为每一位患者的肿瘤单独确定DNA序列可能很快就会成为诊断检查的一部分。就目前来说,这项工作还是实验性的,这个全新的研究领域正在出现显著的成果。

人类的细胞有大约21 000个基因,排列在23对染色体上。如今已为一些肿瘤进行了全部基因的DNA序列与患者的正常DNA之间的比较,结果表明,正常细胞和肿瘤细胞之间的差别微乎其微。平均而言,这类实验大约会显示40到60个异常。换句话说,如果我们把人类基因组看成是一座有23册书(染色体)的图书馆,每册书有大约1 000页(基因),那么整个肿瘤细胞版本"图书馆"的排字错误总共有40到60个。此外,这种基因上的"排印错误"有很多实际上并不会改变基因的"含义",所产生的蛋白质仍然会保留正常的功能。癌症过程的主要驱动因素可以归结为大约12条路径。以这种方式进行研究的癌症中突变或失能的基因都属于这些路径中的一条,看来也的确出现在研究的所有癌症中。该工作为下一阶段的癌症药物研发指明了道路。新一轮的小分子和单克隆主要(但并非全部)关注单一分子,如赫赛汀所针对的HER2。这一新的全基因组研究

76

工作则突出表明有必要以多种基因而非单个成员的路径为目标。未来的药物筛检有可能关注肿瘤生物学的这一方面，与全基因组筛检联手，查明特定肿瘤中关键的突变基因。它也开启了一种可能性，也就是未来的药物将在有特定遗传标记存在的情况下起效。因此，将全基因组测序与诊断联系起来，可以指引人们去寻找肿瘤医学的"圣杯"之一，即药物治疗的个性化选择。

临床前期

新药研发的第一步是为人类研究选择合适的化合物。这日益得益于上文描述的癌症路径研究工作。当前，查找这类化合物可以采取很多形式，从化合物的随机筛检，到定向合成药物，以命中肿瘤细胞中预先明确的异常情况。当前在临床中使用的药物有很多来源，其中有些在上一章已经谈过了。候选药物的初步测试将包括实验室里的肿瘤细胞实验。这些肿瘤细胞有各种来源，从人类的恶性肿瘤到实验室动物产生的人工肿瘤。某些人类细胞系是从手术切除的恶性肿瘤中提取碎片，并在实验室的细胞培养基上培养而来的。这个过程在概念上非常诱人——可以在"真正的"肿瘤上测试药物。

这样的细胞系有很多种，最著名的大概是海拉细胞系了。这个细胞系来自一个名叫海莉耶塔·拉克斯（起初为了保护她的隐私，也曾称其为海伦·莱恩或海伦·拉森）的女人的子宫肿瘤碎片，广泛应用于全世界各地的实验室。顺便提一句，她本人或家属都没有同意或允许这一做法，因此1990年在加州有一次著名的庭审，法庭判决，这样的做法在美国是合法的。英国和其他国家的情况有所不同，如今，根据法律规定，采集组织必须在患者知情的情况下征得其同意方能进行。根据计算，人工培养的海拉细胞比拉克斯女士一生生长的"正常"细胞还要多很多倍，这使得她以一种奇怪的方式得到了永生。然而细胞系的问题在于，大多数试图培养患者肿瘤细胞的努力都以失败告终。因此，我们拥有的细胞系可能缺乏对典型肿瘤的代表性，因为海拉细胞只代表海莉耶塔·拉克斯一个人。然而尽管有这样的局限，人类肿瘤细胞系仍是癌症研究和药物测试的关键组分。

应用的第二种形式的细胞系得自动物肿瘤，大多数来自小鼠。这些肿瘤中有很多都是人为设计的。一个很好的例子就是在前列腺癌研究中使用的一种人工设计的细胞系。小鼠不像人类那样，会患上前列腺癌，但还是有可能识别小鼠前列腺所表达的基因，并利用那些基因的启动子区域（见第二章）来驱动引发肿瘤的蛋白质的产生。在小鼠的例子中，使用的是来自一种名为SV40的致癌病毒的基因，它有一个古怪的名字，叫"大T"。顺带说一下，尽管很多基因的名字都是一连串难记的字母和数字（毕竟单是人类基因就有21 000个——要起名字的非常多），仍有一小部分名字一个（大T）比一个（刺猬、无缺）古怪，还有些有趣透顶——参与细胞发送信号的一对基因被叫作"疯子"和"麦克斯"！

为了让小鼠长出前列腺肿瘤，必须把包含有前列腺特异基因启动子和SV40-T基因的杂合基因插入一个小鼠的受精卵。如果插入成功，就会得到一只转基因小鼠，这样，成长的小鼠就能在其前列腺中表达外来的基因了。可以预测，这些小鼠会继

78

续长出多个前列腺肿瘤。人们培育了一些这种易患癌症的小鼠，该品系被称作"小鼠前列腺转基因腺癌"（TRAMP）模型。事实证明，这些小鼠有多种用途。首先，因为小鼠一定能长出肿瘤，它们可被用于检验诸如饮食干预等预防癌症的策略。其次，它们的肿瘤可以用于测试药物治疗的有效性。最后，来自TRAMP小鼠的肿瘤细胞已经在实验室成功地培养出来，这些细胞系可以供试验使用：既可单独使用，也可被重新移植进同一小鼠品系的成年动物体内——这比等待TRAMP小鼠本身长出肿瘤来要快得多，可复制性也更强。上面的讨论显然又表明，这些模型只能代表人类疾病的某些方面，而不是其完美的复制品。因此，它们虽然有用，但药物最终还是必须在人类身上进行测试。

在一种药物可以施用于人类之前，需要进一步的临床前期测试——毒性试验。尽管动物模型和细胞培养可以作为有用指标，以观察一种药物是否对人有效，但我们无法据此判断该药物是否安全。我们还需要知道是否有望在患者体内施用足以对肿瘤产生实际影响的药物剂量。探究这个问题的标准方法是不断提高给动物群组的剂量，直到开始看到有动物死于药物的副作用为止。还有一些相当可怕的标准措施，如杀死一定比例的试验对象的药物剂量——术语称之为致死剂量（LD）试验。LD50（杀死50%动物的剂量）和LD10（10%的死亡率）等方法得到了广泛应用，也引起了来自反活体解剖组织的许多争议。我并不想探究动物试验本身的伦理——在我看来，这是见仁见智之事。如果你认为此事是不道德的，那么，无论有多少争论一般都不会让你改变立场。不过我确实认为，有必要批判性地考察一下动物试验的科学基础，以便将不必要的痛苦降至最低。LD50 试验有很多显而易见的问题——例如，对于某种给定的化合物来说，LD50 在不同物种之间的差异很大，因此仍会让人类对象面临风险。不过，如果在远低于必要的治疗水平的剂量下，LD50 试验证明毒性很大的化合物不太可能是安全的，也不值得进行人类试验。无论孰是孰非，也不管临床前毒性试验的局限性如何，目前监管当局要求在就某种药物开展任何人类试验之前，这类试验至少要在两个物种上进行，其中一种必须是非啮齿类（例如狗）。

一期试验

研发出候选药物，并完成必要的临床前试验程序之后，下一步就是在人类对象身上进行试验了。从逻辑上讲，这个步骤被叫作一期试验。对于降压药等很多药物而言，这个试验将在"正常"的志愿者身上进行，一般是有报酬的。总的来说，这些人都是健康的青年男子（而不是女人，因为存在对胎儿造成意外伤害的风险）。对于往往毒性很强并有致癌可能的癌症药物而言，这显然不是合适的做法，因而一期试验通常都在那些穷尽了所有标准治疗方案的患者身上进行。一期试验的经典形式是：最初有三位患者接受保守的低剂量治疗并观察其效果。如果没有产生不可接受的毒性，再安排另外三位患者接受更高剂量的治疗，以此类推。显然，大多数药物最终总会达到那个有不可接受的副作用出现的剂量（术语称之为"剂量限制性毒性"，或 DLT）。如果一位患者经历了 DLT，就会有更多的患者接受同等剂量的治疗。如果六位患者中有两名或更多的人经历 DLT，那么就达

到了该药物的"最大耐受剂量"（MTD），试验就此结束。MTD
之下的剂量将会用来做进一步的研究。

经典的一期试验的优点就是操作简单，但显然也有局限性。首先，不同的患者对可能的剂量限制性副作用的易感性不同。如果试验中有太多容易出现副作用的患者，最大耐受剂量的预测值就会过低，反之亦然。其次，并非所有的药物都需要用最大耐受剂量。例如，阻断激素受体的药物只需足够的剂量便可阻断目标。超过此剂量的任何过量施药都只会增加毒性而毫无益处。因此，对于这类药物的试验，就有必要明确规定所需的终点，以避免参与者经受不必要的药物毒性。

一期试验的主要问题与患者的需求有关。在大多数情况下，这些研究都发生在那些穷尽了所有标准治疗方案，显然迫切需要进一步可行疗法的患者身上。就其本质而言，一期试验使用的药物一般低于其可能的治疗范围，因此获益的机会也较低。此外，参与一项研究的最后六位患者中，至少有两位将会接受过高的剂量，经历严重的副作用。最后，进入一期试验的大多数药物都因为无法预见的问题而不能施用足够的剂量，或者干脆对目标肿瘤没有任何疗效，因而实际上无甚治疗价值。因此，大多数患者需要把进入一期试验主要看作是为他人奉献的行为，实际情况也的确如此，参与试验的很多患者会说："好吧，如果这能在我死后帮助其他的人，那也值了。"尽管如此，伦理委员会和医生们仍必须小心保护脆弱绝望的患者免受这些试验的伤害。

二期试验

如果某种药剂在一期中表现出色——换句话说，副作用既

可控也可接受，通常还有证据表明对肿瘤有积极影响，那么接下 81
来就会进入二期试验。二期研究的目标是更详细地研究药效。
药物将以一期确定的最佳剂量进行试验，参与其中的是一群经
评估有可能从中获益的患者。这显然与一期不同，剂量不足或
过量的风险大大减少了，但仍然存在，原因就如上文所述，一期
确定剂量的机制存在着局限性。此外，由于选择患者的依据是有
无可能获益，参与者的风险/获益率要高得多。一般来说，有多达
40或50位患者会进入二期试验，在更加明确、通常也更适合的患
者人群中，最终目标是药物的功效，当然也包括安全性。

　　如何定义药效是个大问题。一般来说，能使肿瘤缩小的药
剂便可被定义为有效，这样就产生了一系列标准化的定义方法，
来定义肿瘤缩小多少才算是值得尝试的反应。最广泛使用的方
法是RECIST（实体瘤临床疗效评价标准）系统，该系统首次发
表于2000年，并在2009年1月进行了更新。疾病应答可以宽泛
地分为如下类别：

- 完全缓解：所有可评估的病灶都消失了；
- 部分缓解：所有可评估的病灶按预先明确的程度而缩
  小了；
- 病情稳定：变化不足以归于另一类别；
- 病情进展：病灶按预先明确的程度恶化，或有新的肿瘤病
  灶出现。

　　这一评估系统的基本原则很简单，实际应用却很复杂。和
很多事情一样，魔鬼就在细节之中——以下是一份（并不全面

第四章　癌症研究

的）棘手问题清单，说明了问题的困难程度：

- 肿瘤应该增长多大才算得上病情进展？
- 它应该缩小多少才算得上对治疗产生了反应？
- 某些肿块缩小而其他肿块却没有，该当如何？
- 何时进行应答测量（太早会报告不足；太晚则患者有可能开始复发）？
- 骨骼或胸膜（肺脏周围的内膜）等组织没有离散的肿块可供测量，如何评估那里的肿瘤病灶？

最后一点是主要感染骨骼的前列腺癌等疾病特有的问题。因此，尽管治疗反应仍是一项重要的药物活性测试，人们如今却越来越多地使用第二组测量方法——其依据是患者需要多长时间病情才会开始恶化，术语称之为"进展时间"。事实证明，这对与肾脏有关的癌症等病的靶向分子新疗法来说尤其重要。这种病的大肿块常常会缩小，但程度低于通常的 RECIST 标准。在复核这些患者的扫描影像时，肿瘤的外观明显改变了，核心部分的"活性"似乎也不如从前——切除肿块后发现中间有坏死组织，就证明了这一点。与此同时，与肿瘤有关的症状往往也得到了改善。因此，对这些患者来说，"稳定"病情的时间延长了，成为一个非常有意义的结果。病情进展的延缓因而经常被用作评估某种药剂活性的方法。最后，当然可以根据对整体存活时间的影响来评估药效。这种方法在二期中不太常被用作主要结果，原因有很多，其中最主要的就是时间——毕竟，最终目标是尽快确定哪些药剂可以进入三期的批准试验。

三期试验

如果某种药剂在二期表现出令人鼓舞的活性，其毒性也可接受，那么就会进入三期试验，将该药剂与当前的治疗标准进行比较。如果该药剂是一种新药，这一般还会涉及制药公司与诸如英国药物和保健产品监管署（MHRA）、欧洲药品管理局（EMA）及美国食品药品监督管理局（FDA）等监管机构一起对试验进行讨论。这些机构会对适当的对照组疗法以及获得批准必须达到的结果给出意见。对照组可能是现有的一种药物或组合药物，也可能是所谓的"最佳支持治疗"。如果没有明确的标准疗法，就会选择后一个选项——患者接受临床医师认为合适的任何缓解措施。

三期试验的标志性特点是，患者的治疗方案是随机分派的。这保证了患者在不同的试验组别之间平均分配，由于预后更好或更坏的患者被集中在一个试验组里而造成结果差异的风险也会被降至最低。虽然这一设计在科学上很有道理，并被视为评估方法的"黄金标准"，但万事均有其局限性。

首先，同时也最明显的是，当对照组是最佳支持治疗或更糟糕的安慰剂药物时，患者会不愿意参与，这是可以理解的。此时显然需要细致的解释和支持，特别是要解释清楚如果没有其他经过证实的替代疗法，那么试验之外的疗法与对照组无异。然而，三期试验常常不是将新药物与安慰剂进行比较，而是与当前标准疗法比较。这在临床上一般更容易解释，因为每个人都接受了治疗，而新药可能不如旧药——这些只有试验完成之后才会知道。就算对照组是安慰剂，这也绝非在假设新药必定更优——药物无异于安慰剂的试验实例有很多，甚至效果更差的例子也不是没有——它可能既有毒性又无药效。

其次，大多数新药只会略强于现有的药物，因而试验各组之间的差异可能会很小。为了检测微小的差异，有必要扩大样本容量，以确保结果在统计学上的置信度。鉴于统计学是一门饱受嘲笑、中伤和误解的科学，用一个简单的例子来说明样本容量为何要大是很有帮助的。假设我们想评估用来抛出的那枚硬币是两面平衡还是有所偏重。如果我们抛了一次，则要么得到正面，要么得到反面（忽略硬币立住的可能性！）。如果我们再抛一次，并得到同样的结果，我们得到（比方说）100%的正面，0%的反面。但根据这样的样本容量没人能说这枚硬币有一面更重。假如我们继续下去，抛了10次——6次正面，4次反面——我们有把握说这枚硬币两面不一样重吗？大概没有。然而，如果我们抛了100次，60次正面，40次反面，或是抛了1 000次，600次正面，400次反面，我们就会越来越有把握说这枚硬币真的有偏重。把问题反过来问就更难了：如果我们得到501次对499次，可以说这枚硬币有偏重吗？大概还是不会。但510次对490次呢？520次对480次又如何？两个数字要有多相近，才可以说差异大概是巧合，而不是因为硬币有偏重？就连600次对400次这样大的差异也可以是一枚公正的硬币发生的巧合，但可能性很低。因此，一个试验的统计方案非常关键，它会明确规定需要多少患者，才能在试验开始前可靠地检测出被认为具有临床重要性的最小差异。对于测试晚期癌症新药的试验来说，至少要按照三个月存活期的平均改善情况来测试。正如我们抛硬币的例子那样，这有可能是碰巧，因此，试验统计学家会计算需要多

癌
症

少患者来可靠地显示（或排除）这种差异——通常（在很大程度上任意地）定义为20次中出现少于1次的偶然结果。

大多数现代试验都会设立一个委员会［通常称作"独立数据监察委员会"（IDMC）或"数据与安全监察委员会"（DSMC）］，独立监察不断累积的结果。该委员会的设置主要是为了保护患者，例如，如果有不可预知的毒性问题，试验会尽早停止。在试验过程的后期，如果提前实现了预先确定的终点，IDMC会终止研究。这样就可以尽快发布数据，也方便其他患者尽早用上这种药物。反过来，IDMC也可能认为试验永远不可能表现出显著的差异，并因其徒劳无益而提早终止试验。

试验的终点充满争议。试验所费不赀，每每在1亿美元以上，因而制药公司希望它们能尽可能规模小、进程快。与此相反，监管者希望有最可靠的结果衡量指标，因而希望延长随访时间或扩大样本规模。社会大众的需求在两者之间。我们都希望有更好的药物，如果患上癌症，恨不得立刻能用上它们。同样，我们也希望它们是安全的。此外，试验的规模越大、时间越长，制药公司为了抵消更高的研发成本，就会提高药价——参见第五章对这个主题的详细讨论。随着卫生预算的增加，降低药价的压力就会上升，使得贫困国家的癌症患者获取新药越来越受限。为了摆脱这种矛盾的紧张关系，研究者日益致力于寻找所谓的"替代"终点，旨在尽早选择一个可以准确预测试验最终结果的终点。二期试验的应答率就是替代终点的一个例子，用于选择一种药物投入三期研究。问题在于，应答率和监管者要求的那种终点（如存活率改善）之间的相关，并没有好到足以让二期的高应答率直接促成药物获批。同样的情况一般也适用于随机试验中应答率之间的比较。

为了避免使用基于存活率的比较（那显然耗时很长），研究者必须证明，某种早期的指标能够可靠地预测最终的结果。上文提到的"延缓进展时间"就是一例。这指的是肿瘤以预先明确的数量生长或扩散所需的时间，通常用来作为早期乳腺癌的调查试验的一个终点。在某些疾病的环境中，例如前列腺癌中的PSA，候选标记并不可靠，前列腺癌的药物目前仍然需要证明存活率有所提高才能获得批准。当前，前列腺癌的研究正在评估一种应答的新方法，即计算循环系统中的肿瘤细胞数量。一般来说，这些数字都极其微小——关键的临界水平是每7.5毫升血液中有大约5个——这就像是在数千万个血细胞的巨大草堆中寻找区区数根缝衣针。当前很多疾病像前列腺癌一样，被困在整体存活率的终点前，如果这样的检测获得了批准，就可以大大加快癌症药物研发的步伐。因为试验时间缩短，成本更低，获得批准后，同样也会降低药物的价格。

现有治疗的比较

上文描述的一期到三期的方案可以广泛地适用于任何新技术或新药物的组合，然而，不同国家的要求也各不相同。现有药物新组合的比较试验往往是由英国癌症研究中心或美国国家癌症研究所这样的学术组织进行的。使用上面的模板会得到能够影响实践的可靠结果，一般来说也是推进医疗实践的黄金标准。但这个系统在手术技术、放疗设备、其他设备以及生物标记物等方面的明确性就差多了。例如，机器人手术等新技术是作为渐进式改进事物被引入的。这些"改进"被看作是不言而喻的，而实际上或许根本不是那回事。例如,将开放式手术与机器人辅助手术进行比较:进入身体的途径就不相同;外科医生的双手与组织之间的触觉联系在机器人辅助手术中消失了;止血或肠穿孔等并发症或许会引发不同程度的风险,可能需要从机器人辅助转换到开放式的传统手术上来;外科医生在培训的情况下,手术时间可能会更长,如此等等。显然,这些因素中的每一个都完全有可能对结果产生重大影响。此外,还有成本的大问题。一台手术机器人的成本超过100万英镑,每年还需要10万到15万英镑的运营成本。就算结果更好一些,比方说出院时间提前一些,又值得付出多少代价呢?

人们或许以为在例如前列腺切除手术中采用这样的技术也有同样的试验要求,就像前列腺癌新药的研发所需的试验那样,而结果一样或更好。但这样的试验从未进行过,而外科机器人已经在全世界各大手术中心运作起来了,尤其是在美国。为何存在这样巨大的差异呢?本质上,新设备只需在其设计目的上表现出安全性与适用性即可。在变化的确很小并且是渐进式改进的情况下,进行一次大型试验来证明一种新的手术刀略好一些,这种做法显然不切实际,大概也毫无意义。变化在某个时间点就不再是渐进式的了,在我看来,手术机器人正是这方面的一个好例子,而我们仍把这些机器人看作一种稍有改善的手术刀。特别是在美国,购买一台手术机器人成为医院营销的重要噱头:它是一种标志性的工具,哪个开拓进取的机构不想拥有它呢?在医疗系统为成本上升焦头烂额之际,解决这个问题很可能变得越来越重要。当然,可以想见,新技术实际上节约了成本。坚持使用机器人,声称学习过程缩短,住院天数变少,并发症发生率降低可以抵消投入资金和运营成本,这种说法并非不合情理。然而,就目前而言,我们还是不甚清楚。

类似的争论也适用于成像和其他诊断检查。同样,这里也有一个显而易见之事无须研究证明的问题:成像更加清晰的扫描很可能比模糊的好!然而,仔细考察就会发现,实际情况更加复杂。比方说,影响决策的一个关键因素是肿瘤是否已扩散到某个特定的器官。一般来说,如果某个已知有风险区域的扫描显示不正常,这很可能代表疾病存在。然而反之并非如此:扫描结果为阴性可能意味着阴性,也可能意味着疾病低于检测阈值。这已经由第三章讨论的假设肝脏扫描说明。这种问题的一个好例子是在淋巴结处检测肿瘤。由于淋巴结是正常的组织,而淋巴结里的肿瘤与正常组织的密度相近(因此成像的外观也相近),所以成像只能告诉我们淋巴结的大小是正常还是异常——

88

癌

症

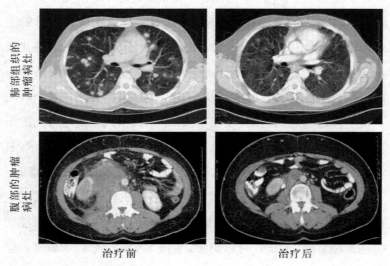

肺部组织的肿瘤病灶

腹部的肿瘤病灶

治疗前　　　　　　　　　治疗后

图22　扫描影像上肿瘤应答的示例

通常来说，临界尺寸是5毫米左右。显然，如果有一个4毫米的肿瘤病灶占据了大部分淋巴结，那么它看起来就会很"正常"。

假设为淋巴结疾病研发出了一种更好的成像检查，该如何评估它呢？这样的检查会与外科设备同属一种监管方法：需要证明其针对所要达到的目的是否安全和适用。安全性一目了然——一期和二期的常规路线显然就很奏效，但我们如何证明"目的适用性"呢？答案是某种形式的临床试验，但终点的问题非常复杂——我们需要检测出多少个含有小型恶性肿瘤的"正常"淋巴结才算有价值呢？可以错过多少个？如何评估"真"阳性率和"真"阴性率？是否该转向更广泛的临床结果，而不是计算淋巴结的数量——比方说，与标准的治疗方式相比，这项检查的应用是否会导致更好的临床结果，例如患者的存活时间更长了？

在新扫描仪器的购置成本非常高的情况下，在成像技术上，这些也都是非常麻烦的问题。就连对新的造影剂这种加强现有扫描仪器的技术来说，这些问题也很严重，全球对此都没有一致的单一解决方案。

类似的争论也适用于诊断检查。同样，乍看之下，问题似乎很简单——如果有一种血液检查与癌症相关，就应该把它作为临床决策的基础之一。但如果我们查阅文献，就会发现有很多检查都与疾病存在与否相关，但鲜有在实际中用于临床的——何以至此？关于这个问题，最主要的答案是该检查必须对已知的内容给出额外的信息。例如，有大量的尿液检查与膀胱癌相关，但英国没有使用其中的任何一个。膀胱癌疑似患者需要做膀胱镜检查来确认诊断。可用的尿液检查不够可靠，不足以让患者免于膀胱镜检查。一旦检查了膀胱，如果发现肿瘤，就需要活组织检查。同样，这些检查的可靠性也不足以排除活检的需要。此外，切除活检也是治疗的一部分，因此无论这项检查有多优秀，患者仍需手术。预后的判断如何呢？同样，尿液检查很好，但又不像被切除肿瘤的病理学研究那么好，所以它还是没有给出额外信息。鉴于以上所述，诊断过程的检查适用与否在于它对结果的影响——该项检查是否可以免去侵入性治疗，或预测哪些治疗方案是最佳的？这需要进行大规模试验，就像为药物获批而进行的那些，也解释了为什么辅助临床决策的既有检查或标记物少之又少。

有不少标记物与疾病密切相关，可以在出现临床症状或扫描结果发生明显变化之前，用来预测临床事件。这样的标记物包括前列腺癌中的PSA、卵巢癌中的CA125，以及睾丸癌中的AFP和HCG等等。就算存在良好的标记物，也不一定能用它们来取代其他的临床评估方法。例如，尽管PSA的变化大致能够反映病情的变化，可以影响临床结果的某些治疗（名为双膦酸盐类的骨骼强化药物就是一个很好的例子），对PSA含量的影响却很小，虽说它有助于防止癌症对骨骼造成损伤。更加惊人的是，最近对卵巢癌和标记物作用进行的一次大规模研究得出了非常反直觉的结果。血液中CA125含量的上升准确预测了临床上的复发。人们或许以为尽早治疗复发会比等到症状发展时再治疗要好。该研究比较了标记物驱动型治疗的策略（就是标记物含量一旦升高，就开始对复发进行治疗）与临床上的症状驱动型治疗。总共有大约1 500名女性参与了这项研究，在检测更严密的女性中更早地采取治疗并未影响其存活时间。更惊人的是，接受临床驱动型治疗的女性，其生活质量和焦虑程度更好一些——因此，密切检测和早期治疗的总体效果实际上较差。

当前研究的一大焦点是个体化治疗，也就是识别标记物，从而根据个人的具体情况来调整治疗。描述肿瘤特点的方式有很多——通过其DNA的突变、蛋白质表达的模式、观察各种酶的活性等等。然而，尽管识别与不同结果相关的模式相对容易，但从以上讨论中可以明显看出，这并不足以改变治疗。为了证明其临床价值，需要临床试验将候选的标记物驱动型策略与标准的治疗方法进行比较。正如上文卵巢癌的例子所表明的那样，就算有优秀的标记物也无法确保一定能得到期待的结果。可能会出现的另一个问题是，正在研发中的候选标记物数量可能超出了研究团队进行试验的能力，甚或多出很多倍。此外，标记物实际上把一种疾病从一种同质体变成了彼此不同的若干子实体。因为优秀的试验需要大量参与者，这使得进行试验变得更加困难，因为该疾病实际上变得更加罕见了。肾癌最近出现的变化可以证明这一点。不久前，研究者描述了一些病理上的变体，但在靶向小分子出现之前，这些变体并未给治疗方案带来什么影响。如上文讨论的那样，肾透明细胞癌的异常情况（约占总数的70%）催生了新的治疗方法。那么剩下的30%该当如何？这30%是由几种不同的亚型组成的，因为每一种都实在罕见，试验如今变得困难起来。结果，我们实际上不清楚该如何处理这些亚型。这些所谓的"孤儿"疾病会越来越常见，并且因为试验数据对指导治疗用处不大而问题重重，试验也因为人数不够而困难起来。

结　语

　　接下来的几年，我们将会在癌症新药、新的生物标记物，以及诸如手术机器人等激动人心并充满未来感的技术上迎来很多令人振奋的进展。如何将这些发展融入实践中，在很大程度上依赖于支撑它们使用的临床研究。然而，新技术往往尤其会通过营销而非试验的渠道来推广。在医疗保健预算面临着人口老龄化和信贷紧缩带来的巨额债务的压力下，我们如何批准、监管和资助这些设备将会越来越问题重重。

92

癌
症

癌症治疗的经济因素

前面几章说明了现代癌症治疗极其复杂的性质,以及医学技术和药物疗法日新月异的发展。如上一章所述,这些变化得益于药物生产商和医疗设备制造商对新疗法的巨大投资。显然,新疗法必须收取回报,一般来说,成本也高于它们所取代的旧疗法。也有一些例外的情况,例如,一种提高治愈率的治疗方法可以降低后续疗法的下游开支,因而可能会使所使用的医疗资源净减少。衡量这些相互依存的变化显然非常复杂,因此,很多医疗保健的经济决策都关注新技术的直接购置成本(这些很容易衡量),而不是次级的下游变化。癌症治疗经常发生的情况是,这些成本都集中在生命的终点附近,从而引发充满争议的经费难题。本章用部分篇幅讨论了不同的医疗保健系统是如何应对这些难题的。

相比于单个药物的成本,经济因素对癌症治疗的显著影响也更多体现在宏观经济的层面上。总体而言,世界上的发达经济体有全面的医疗保健系统,广泛覆盖了从摇篮到坟墓的健康 93

91

问题。不同的系统各有其优缺点，但主要的差别存在于发达世界与欠发达世界之间。显然，如果缺乏基础设施，对大多数人来说，就根本无须讨论是否要购买某种昂贵的新药。可以预测一下这些影响的规模：图23显示了人均国民生产总值（pcGNP）与以岁数计算的预期寿命之间的相互影响。可以看到有一些收入非常低的国家，其预期寿命不出所料也很低。然而，还有一些国家的pcGNP低于每年1 000美元，但预期寿命却超过了65岁。这些国家包括埃及、特立尼达以及中国。它们的共同特点是有一个综合公共卫生系统和良好的围产期保健。与此相反，还有些国家的pcGNP超过了2 000美元，而预期寿命却低于60岁。问题似乎在于HIV的感染率较高。因而笼统地说，一个国家的富裕程度会影响医疗保健的质量和预期寿命，这不足为奇，但其他因素也会起到重要的作用。其中一些因素很容易受到政府可控要素的影响，例如为实现各类资源和公共卫生活动等的影响最大化的整体布局。相反，在这个分布的顶端，国民收入一旦达到某个水平，就没有多少进步的空间了，预期寿命显然在接近80岁的位置达到上限。至于这种情况是否会在未来随着技术改善而变化，仍有待观察。

如果我们继续考察国民收入对癌症的影响，就会看到另一个有趣的结果。随着财富的增加，患癌的风险也在增加。这部分归因于预期寿命延长的影响——如果你没有饿死或是年纪轻轻便死于感染，就有大得多的机会能活到相对较大的年纪，患上癌症。其他因素也起到了作用，例如，一旦国民收入超过人均5 000美元，癌症的发生率就会达到每年每10万人中250—400例（见图24）。然而，有一些国家的国民收入在此范围之内，但癌症发生率却低于此值的三分之一，这些国家都在中东地区。这归因于尽管国民收入有所提高，他们却普遍遵守更传统、非西化的生活方式。与之相反，有一组国家的癌症发生率和西方一样高，国民收入却低于每人5 000美元。这些前苏联阵营的国家乍看之下似乎结果最糟——患有西方的疾病，收入却属于发展中世界。然而细察之下，情况却没有那么悲观——低收入诚然不假，但高癌症率却是因为有着组织完善的医疗保健系统，他们的预期寿命较长。近来关于"公费医疗"优缺点的讨论，特别是关于英国国家医疗服务体系（NHS）和美国系统的讨论，都强调有必要进行冷静客观的分析。尽管美英两国的某些结果确实存在差别，但在医疗保健系统高度发达的所有国家，整体预期寿命

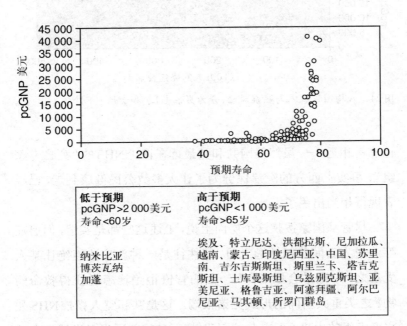

低于预期	高于预期
pcGNP>2 000美元	pcGNP<1 000美元
寿命<60岁	寿命>65岁
纳米比亚	埃及、特立尼达、洪都拉斯、尼加拉瓜、
博茨瓦纳	越南、蒙古、印度尼西亚、中国、苏里
加蓬	南、吉尔吉斯斯坦、斯里兰卡、塔吉克
	斯坦、土库曼斯坦、乌兹别克斯坦、亚
	美尼亚、格鲁吉亚、阿塞拜疆、阿尔巴
	尼亚、马其顿、所罗门群岛

图23　人均国民总收入和预期寿命

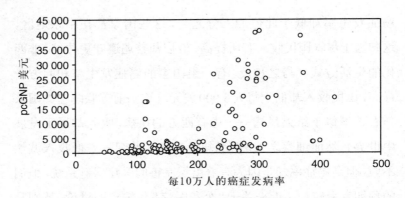

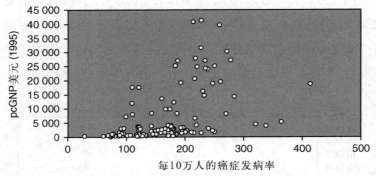

图24　人均国民收入与癌症风险,分为男性(上)和女性(下)

也非常相近——虽然美国共和党最近在谈论NHS的"死亡专家组",事实上西方的医疗保健为了让大多数公民健康到老,已经表现得相当出色了。

尽管从国家拨款这个层面上说,上述这些都是实情,但癌症疗法成为新闻热门话题之日,却往往是一种新疗法拒绝让某人受惠之时,通常会以《千人一面的官僚拒绝让患者获得救命药96 物》之类重大新闻的形式见诸报端。这是共和党人指控NHS死亡专家组的由来(事实上,没有医疗保健的美国患者当然也会被另一套官僚或银行经理拒绝他们使用同一种疗法）。为什么在这些世上最富裕的国家会发生这样的事情？经费和成本可能的未来趋势又会怎样？

和大多数商品一样，医疗成本也会年复一年地上升，也就是通货膨胀。医疗的通胀率是可以衡量的，一般来说，它会高于整个国家的基本通胀率。这一点很重要，因为它意味着如果不削减成本，久而久之，医疗保健为了与新技术同步，会消耗掉更高比例的国民收入。美国就是最好的证明：2008年，美国的医疗通胀率是6.9%，大概是该国其他通胀率的两倍。根据当前的预测，这会导致美国的医疗卫生支出从2008年占国民收入的17%上升到2017年的占比20%。自金融危机以来，世界经济的巨大变化让这种情况难以为继。类似的数字也适用于全世界各大经济体。成本为何会以这种方式上升？要知道在NHS创建之初，该机构的主要设计师之一安奈林·贝文曾展望，因为健康的改善，成本会随着时间的推移而下降。原因在于研发新疗法的成本。为某种癌症疗法获批而进行的一次试验通常会花费大约1亿英镑。因此，新获批的药物需要收回这些庞大的研发成本，外加在此过程中以失败告终，因而根本不会产生任何效益的所有药物的成本。在药物获批之时剩余的专利期限通常是10年或更短，因为药物在获批过程完成的多年之前就需要保护专利了。因此，一种新药的大部分成本反映的都是获批前发生的成本——而实际生产尽管昂贵，通常却只占每一粒药价格的一小部分。一种药的专利到期后，在仿制药的竞争之下，其价格通常会下跌90%—95%，就反映了这一点。

因此，一种新药的要价，会与收回庞大的研发成本以及在

97

专利许可到期之前的盈利密切相关。随着全球化的发展，全世界的价格趋于相近，使得穷国特别难以负担新药的价格。制药公司的定价策略不属于公共领域的问题，但想必是为了在全世界实现收入最大化。对于英国、澳大利亚和新西兰这样的国家来说，这样的定价往往超出了卫生系统准备支付的价格。也有限制较少的卫生系统愿意支付较高的价格，制药公司由此获得的高收入大概会抵消上述卫生系统支付价格的不足。比如在法国，一旦某种药物获批，相关专家均可任意开处方，没有直接的支出上限。这对使用率和总支出都有着巨大的影响，本章后文将谈到这一点。然而，持续的医疗通胀趋势和研发成本的上升将会对世界各地的预算施加压力，让获取治疗变得越来越困难。医疗设备方面也有类似的争论，上一章讨论的机器人手术的新技术就是一例。

位于赫尔辛基备受推崇的卡罗林斯卡学院①最近的一份报告详细调查了癌症药物经费的问题。该报告考察了整个欧盟的趋势，比较了各成员国的支出模式，并总结了全世界的问题。从全球范围来看，2006年的癌症药物市场价值340亿美元，在2008年上升到430亿美元，制药业每年的研究开支为60亿—80亿美元，美国国家癌症研究所另外投入36亿美元，欧盟也追加投入14亿欧元。全世界正在试验的所有药物中，大约有半数是治疗癌症的。在欧盟，每10万人口的癌症药物销售额从1996年的不足50万欧元，上升到了2007年的逾250万欧元——10年中增加到原来的6倍。此外，尽管新药带给预算的压力越来越大，上述

---

① 经查，该学院位于瑞典首都斯德哥尔摩市，原文应有误。——译注

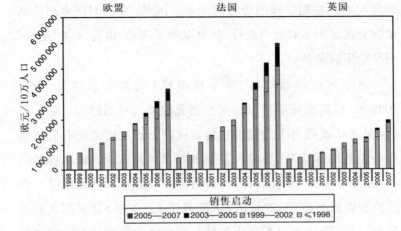

图25 1998—2007年欧盟癌症药物的销售额

药物销售额的增加却并非由于新药的价格昂贵，而主要是因为现有药物的使用与日俱增。图25表明了这两个趋势，显示出按照药物获得批准的年度划分，药物开销的逐年增加。该图还显示了英法两国的对比，法国对肿瘤药物的处方基本上没有控制，而英国则对此严格监管。

　　已有药物的开支为什么会有这样大的增长？答案在于药物获批的过程及随后使用的方式。查看第三章图18关于癌症治疗的分类说明，就可以发现，有大约40%的患者在某个阶段发展成晚期癌症，其中大多数人最终都死于该病。新药最初一般都是在这群患者身上进行试验的，他们患上了不治之症，选择极其有限。例如在乳腺癌中，只有少数患者死于该病，因此，一种新近获批的终末期药物的开支也相对有限。然而，如果某种药物在这个群体中效果良好，那么对于那些有望治愈，但初步治疗后复发风险很高的早期患者，它的表现往往更好。这一群体约占最终会发展为晚期疾病的患者的一半。因此，成功的终末期药物试验会在这些患者身上进行，如果取得了成功，该药就会"迁移"到早期疾病患者中。

　　这个过程在赫赛汀（曲妥珠单抗）的故事里可见一斑。2002年，该药被证明可以延长晚期乳腺癌的存活时间。从一开始，赫赛汀就吸引了大量的宣传。这种新的治疗方法在乳腺癌患者中间迅速成名，导致大量患者要求参加试验。需求如此之大，以至于不得不为感兴趣的合格患者设置试验入组抽签。该药物获得批准后，它的价格（大约每年3万英镑）让英国人觉得高不可及，于是不得不开始在另一组女性中间进行另一种形式的抽签——英国癌症基金的邮政编码抽奖。后来由女性发起的声势浩大的运动成功地推翻了这些限制，但也为其他希望获得昂贵疗法的群体开了先例，这些疗法至今仍在折磨着各国采购当局，英国当局尤感万分为难。

　　2006年在早期疾病中的后续试验表明，如果给术后的早期高风险疾病的女性患者服用赫赛汀，和以前的疗法相比，疾病复发率会降低大约一半。因此，赫赛汀的许可证在同一年扩展到早期疾病患者中。遗憾的是，当前无法识别出哪些患者在手术和放疗后会复发。因为早期高风险组中的大多数女性通过标准疗法已经治愈，有资格接受该药治疗的人数大大增加（在英国增加了约三倍）——存在风险的所有患者都必须接受治疗，而不仅仅是那些注定会复发的人。在女性患者的宣传运动之后，在NHS，符合条件的所有患者都可以获得这种药物。

　　因此，医疗保健系统该如何就新疗法做出决策呢？假设有一种新疗法要花费30 000英镑，并可以把存活期延长6个月，从

- 30 000英镑
- 30 000英镑减去它所取代的疗法费用
- 30 000英镑减去它所取代的疗法费用,再减去其他支持性治疗所节省的费用

　　没有正确答案——这取决于谁来买单,买的是什么。答案一是患者的花费,如果医疗保健系统不能报销这种疗法的话。英国有时就是这样,NHS对它会购买的药物做了限制。旧的标准疗法可以报销,但新药则不能。在基于保险的系统中,额外的药物不在保险覆盖的报销体系之内,这也日益成为患者面临的问题。答案二是提供专家治疗的医院的费用,而医院对每个患者的预算是固定的(NHS的医院正是如此,美国的某些管理式医疗系统也是这样)。答案三是为患者的整个治疗提供资金的组织的价格:可能是NHS或保险公司等机构背后的国家。那么这就引发了另一个问题:相关费用中具体包括了哪些项目?比方说,每当患者死亡,临终关怀的费用大概都差不多。然而,如果像例子中一样,存活时间变长,它们就会属于另一个财政年度的药费支出——这些支出必须要推迟多长时间才可以算作节省?能够提高治愈率的治疗尤其如此,因为这样的支出会推迟到多年之后。同样,这些问题都没有一个简单的答案——不同的医疗保健系统会以不同的方式来解决这些难题。值得考察一下公共卫生专家和保险公司在决定是否资助某个特定疗法时,使用的是哪一种方法。

　　一个常用的方法是预测新疗法所带来的额外寿命的年均成本。对额外生命整体质量的一项调整也常常被用到。目标是产生一种叫质量调整生命年（QALY）的衡量方法。例如，一种治疗延长了一年的寿命，但生命质量降低了50%，将被计为0.5个质量调整生命年。这看上去相当简洁，医疗保健的购买者也可以用它来在不同的疗法之间进行比较：一种药物疗法可以延长三个月的寿命，另一种髋关节置换术能够改善生命质量，却无法延长预期寿命。对于手术和放疗这些成熟的疗法来说，患者常常可以痊愈，因而这种费用会分摊在所增加寿命的一个大数字上。如此说来，尽管大手术很昂贵，在大多数情况下，分摊到每个质量调整生命年的费用却非常低。相反，那些能够稍微延长终末期疾病患者存活时间的新药，其费用与质量调整生命年之比往往非常高，而问题就出在这里，下文将具体说明。

　　调整生命质量所面临的紧迫问题显而易见——我们如何定义一个人的生命质量受到了多少影响？例如，A先生的生活以久坐为主，他喜欢的娱乐方式是看电视，因此某个缺陷如果让他无法奔跑，妨碍不大。但B先生是个铁人三项运动爱好者，如果像A先生那样行动不便会让他非常痛苦。显然，任何质量调整都是主观的，并取决于具体受到影响的人。但无论如何，必须设法得到某种平均值，并把它加到这个等式里去。

　　第二个问题是如何衡量存活的收益。这看起来或许简单直接，但获取批准的试验往往只关注病情恶化所需的时间（即所谓的"进展时间"——见第四章），而不是总体的存活时间。因此，后续的"补救"治疗或许改善了患者起初在试验对照组里的结果。这些试验的终点是由美国食品药品监督管理局和欧洲药品管理局等监管当局设定的，并决定一家公司是否会获得产品上市许可证。然而，仅仅因为某种药物可以上市，并不意味着会有医疗保健系统来采购它。

为了解释这个过程具体如何运作，我们来纵览一下一种治疗晚期肾癌的新药近期进行的试验。在试验中，服用安慰剂的患者病情恶化的速度是服用索拉非尼的患者的两倍。该试验的独立数据监察委员会基于伦理的立场决定，研究应当终止，仍然存活的安慰剂组患者都接受了新药的治疗。后来在分析整体存活时间时，起初服用新药的患者比那些起初服用安慰剂的活得更长。但因为患者从安慰剂改服活性药物的补救效果，新药的存活优势远小于当初由该药对进展时间的影响得出的预期。由于伦理上不允许用不治疗的组别来重复这个试验，因此根本无法计算索拉非尼对晚期肾癌的生存效益。如此一来，该病的每个治疗调整生命年的费用估计也就存在着双重缺陷：对生命质量的影响是主观的，而真正的生存收益不得而知。这种双重不确定性使得英国对肾癌的决策过程从2006年到2009年一度陷入了停滞。

基于质量调整存活时间的决策，是由一家英国机构率先广泛使用的，这家机构有一个奥威尔式的名字，叫作国家健康与临床优化研究所，通常简写为NICE。这个机构旨在为公共卫生服务提供建议，建议后者应该为患者采购哪些疗法，而哪些疗法物非所值，不应定期拨款。NICE不考虑未获批准的或实验性的治疗。一些其他的欧洲国家也采纳了类似的方法，但到目前为止，更偏爱自由市场模式的美国避开了这种集中管控的路线。从最初批准某种药物到提供建议，NICE通常要花费数月甚至数年的时间。在英国，NHS的拨款由"采购商"和"供应商"两者平分。当前，采购商被称作初级保健信托（PCTs），负责在本地做出相同的决策（是否购买某种特定的疗法）。2011年，也就是本书撰写之时，即将到来的NHS改革将把这个采购商角色转移到家庭医生（全科医生）身上。目前的PCTs能力不同，细致程度也有异，他们履行这个角色时往往只提供最廉价的选择，等到NICE后来直接参与指导了，他们才被迫提供较为昂贵的疗法。这继而又导致了无人不晓（臭名昭著）的英国邮政编码抽奖——因为PCTs是基于地理位置的，获得任何NHS的治疗都取决于患者的地址和当地PCTs的决策过程。2008年，这导致花费最高的PCTs在接受癌症治疗的每位患者身上平均分配大约15 000英镑，而花费最低的PCTs为每位患者仅分配大约5 000英镑。比方说在我自己的诊所里，邮政编码在伯明翰（高开支地区）的患者可以轻松获得最新的肾癌药物。相反，大多数周边郡的癌症药物开支相对较低，获取同样的药物受到了极大限制。由于患者显然会在候诊室里交谈，所产生的沮丧和愤怒也就可想而知了。我们在自己的晚期肾癌患者中间按照邮编进行过一次生存时间审查。来自低开支地区的患者平均存活时间约为7—8个月，而来自高开支的伯明翰地区的患者则是大约两年——这是个非常真实而值得关注的差异。此外，被拒绝使用昂贵药物的患者，因为癌症未得到治疗所引起的疾病并发症发病率上升，去医院就诊的次数大约是对照组的三倍。从2006年（新的肾癌药物首次获得批准的年份）开始，这种状况持续了三年，直到2009年初，NICE最终建议将这批药物中的舒尼替尼提供给所有的肾癌患者（但获取其他新近获批的肾癌药物仍然受到严格

癌症

的限制）。显然，未给这些药物拨款的PCTs认为，他们把这笔钱用在其他地方，可以为不同的患者群体产生更大的收益。但是，我没有看到任何可靠证据可以表明，与周边郡县相比，伯明翰缺乏资金的其他患者群体出现了什么较差的结果。因此，我认为当前的英国系统臃肿笨重，充满了不必要的官僚主义，并且在很多情况下耳目闭塞。那些声称代表公众的决策者无法以任何方式为其决策公开负责——比方说，他们并不是通过选举而上台的——也往往不会公开为自己的决策辩护。另一方面，在成本上升、人口老化、预算缩减的时代，必须做出某种形式的取舍，因而像NICE这样的机构大概会在未来风行全世界。

英国拟议中的新采购计划意味着一个群体，即全科医生，将既是采购商也是供应商，而第二个群体，医院的专科护理部门，将会是纯粹的供应商。这意味着如果能把患者拦在医院大门之外，在经济上对全科医生联合体有利，也许是件好事，也许不是。另一方面，他们必须向自己的病人证明他们为什么选择拒绝出资购买某些疗法，因为他们不可避免地必须如此，而当前的PCTs则没有这么做。较低的管理成本是否有可能像政府希望的那样，转化为更好的第一线治疗，仍有待观察，因为在我看来，全科医生为何是决定专科护理选择的最佳人选，还不甚清楚。

与其他类似的欧洲国家相比，英国缓慢复杂的决策过程也会推迟癌症新药的采用，并降低整体的开支。尽管并未正式公布，但据估计，每增加一个质量调整生命年，NICE的目标开支为最多30 000英镑，花费更高的治疗会被拒绝拨款。其他国家采用的方法没有这么形式化，但似乎非正式地应用了更高的临界额度。正因为这一临界点较低，当前英国在癌症药物上的开销

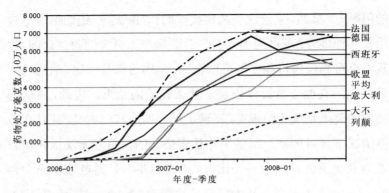

图26 药物舒尼替尼在欧盟的使用

是法德等国限额的大约60%。这一差别似乎特别集中在癌症疗法上，因为在心血管疾病或精神病治疗这另外两大开支领域中，并不存在这样悬殊的差别。治疗肾癌的舒尼替尼在2006年获得批准以来的开支模式很好地说明了这一点，与欧盟的平均值，特别是意大利、法国、德国和西班牙的具体数字相比，英国用于该药的开支上升得既迟又缓（图26）。与我们的欧洲邻国相比，英国的癌症药物开支相对较低，在每个患者身上的开支根据邮编而存在巨大差异，难怪在这个国家观察到的癌症治疗效果相对较差。

开支的未来趋势看来也充满了挑战。英国目前有77种获批的癌症治疗药物（这里忽略了那些支持性治疗的药物）。其中有大约25种是在1995—2005年间获批的。2007—2012年间据估计有50种药物在申请获批。显然，这些药物不是每一个都能成功地越过最后一道关卡。此外，与替代治疗方案相比，很多药物所能提供的收益很小。然而，其中的一些（或许很多）药物可以提供巨大的后续收益。另外，会出现这样的持续趋势，即现有的昂贵新药迁移到早期疾病环境和更大的市场中，就像上文提到用于乳腺癌的赫赛汀的例子那样。这一切无疑会给所有的医疗卫生经济体带来更沉重的财政压力。我参加的国际会议有一个有趣的动向，就是关于这些观点的讨论。直到最近，因为获取新药相对困难，这在英国还只是一个大家感兴趣的话题而已。现在情况愈演愈烈，就连美国的发言人也开始讨论新疗法的可承受性了，而美国此前的医疗预算显然是个无底洞。贝拉克·奥巴马的医改方案也把同样的问题牢牢地提上了美国主流政治议程。

还有一些趋势有可能会缓解压力。首先，过了专利保护期的老药通常会价格暴跌，跌幅往往会高达95%。其次，如果结果的改善幅度足够大，其他医疗成本可能会有补偿性的节省，尽管开支是当下发生的，而节省会较晚且难以追踪（甚或会归于另一个医疗供应商）。最后，更好的疾病行为预测指标或许可以让我们针对那些最有可能获益的人群施用昂贵的疗法。例如，如果我们知道哪些乳腺癌患者只靠手术便可治愈（大多数人），就可以省下很大比例的辅助疗法药物的费用。因此，对于这种预测生物标记物的研究正是当前癌症研究中最热门的领域之一。对临床试验新方法的研究也许同样有助于缩短研发时间，并进而降低药物的成本。

结　语

这些因素在未来会如何起作用仍有待观察，世界各地可能会出现不同的解决方案。在欧洲，我们可能会看到全民享受最先进医疗服务的原则日益陷入困境。在英国，尽管NICE经历了种种运营问题，但该机构根据负担能力做决策的做法可能成为更加普遍的模式。这就引出了与之相关的追加经费问题，这已经是英国的政治难题了。利用私人保险来补足国家供给可能也会变成常态，因为与旨在替代国家供给的政策相比，这样做的成本要低得多。在美国，部分覆盖仍是一个大问题。就算是对有保险的人，我怀疑也会开始尝试对最昂贵的癌症疗法限制开支。在主要的西方国家之外，随着经济的发展和预期寿命的延长，癌症发病率可能会上升。就像本章和上一章所述，最超值的癌症疗法是手术和放疗，而在发展中国家，这些服务可能会越来越多。药物疗法的额外收益相对较小，因此，获得这些药物很可能更多局限于价格较低的老药，而在这些国家，最昂贵的疗法将仅限于少数人。

107

108

癌
症

癌症治疗的替代和补充方法

　　研究表明，至少有半数的癌症患者在常规医学之外还求助于补充或替代医学（有人怀疑，余下的人群中还有很多根本没有告诉我们）。这些医学的形式各式各样，包括少数族裔患者使用的传统疗法。尽管"补充"和"替代"这两个词有时可以互换使用，但还是应该区分一下所谓主流医疗之外的这两种不同的方法。因此，我会把那些旨在以支持的形式与常规疗法同时进行的称为补充医学。芳香疗法就是一例，它在根本上与患者继续其常规疗法并不冲突。实际上，芳香疗法有助于提高治疗依从性，或是降低对泻药或止痛药等额外药物的需求。除了芳香疗法等准医学疗法之外，主流医疗保健和其他"治疗师"还会提供针灸和顺势疗法等治疗。另一方面，替代医学旨在取消主流疗法，代之以常规医学认为在最好的情况下也不过是未经检验，在最糟的情况下还可能是有害的疗法。在实践中，不可能把各种治疗严格地归类为补充疗法或替代疗法，因为一个患者可能会在接受常规治疗的同时使用某种药物或疗法，而另一个患者可 109

能会用同样的药物或疗法来取代常规治疗——区别在于意图和内容,两者兼而有之。

世上有大量的替代和补充医学,彼此各不相同,包括顺势疗法、针灸、各种饮食疗法、草药、芳香疗法,还有诸如水晶疗法、观想,以及少数族裔使用的传统疗法等等。对这些疗法一一详细分析超出了本书的范围,因此我会尝试选择一些例子,来总结一下补充和替代疗法与癌症治疗之间的相互作用和影响。在此之前,可以来感受一下这些疗法的使用范围之广、规模之大。虽说各国情况不同,但它们在美国的使用或许能够代表发达世界的普遍情形。由于美国的开支很容易量化,我会分类讲解美国国立卫生研究院提供的近期数据。标题数字显示,2007年,8 800万美国人在补充或替代医学上花费达339亿美元之巨。这在美国的全部自费医疗开支中占比超过10%。此外还有230亿美元花在了维生素和矿物质补充剂上。考虑到美国公民面对的巨额医疗账单,他们会另外花这么一大笔钱,显然非常惊人。按照2007年的汇率,这可以为整个英国人口提供大约六个月的医疗保健。这些数字显然与总支出有关,而不只是由癌症患者花的钱;然而,它们的确能让人真切感受到这些治疗的使用范围之广。类似的开销存在于所有的工业化国家。这些可是世界上教育最发达的国家,如前所述,它们一般都会提供医疗保健服务,让大多数人得以活到老年,那么为什么它们的公民会花费如此巨额的钱款在额外治疗上,其中大多数根本未经证明?显然,在不太富裕的国家,部分人口或许只能负担得起传统疗法,因而可能是不同的力量在起作用。

在继续讨论这个问题之前,有必要仔细研究一下钱到底花在了什么地方。我还是会使用美国的数字，虽说其他地方的分摊方式可能不大一样，但我认为，这可以让我们感受到人们想要的到底是什么。如果我们能够理解这一点，或许就有助于解释上面的矛盾。

美国报告中最大的一类是"非维生素、非矿物质的天然产品"。这些想必是各种各样的草药——上文已经提到，在大约230亿美元的维生素补充剂和硒等矿物质的开支中，**不包括**这一项。还有41亿美元花在专注心理健康的技术上，无论其内容是否包括像瑜伽这样的运动。显然，这些是否真的该归于此类还值得商榷，因为个人的动机很明确——这让他们感觉良好。这本身显然就是一个好处，我觉得再讨论下去就没什么必要了。同样的理由也适用于花在身心放松技术上的2亿美元开支。

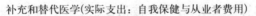
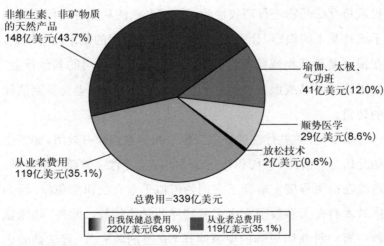

补充和替代医学(实际支出：自我保健与从业者费用)

非维生素、非矿物质
的天然产品
148亿美元(43.7%)

瑜伽、太极、
气功班
41亿美元(12.0%)

顺势医学
29亿美元(8.6%)

放松技术
2亿美元(0.6%)

从业者费用
119亿美元(35.1%)

总费用=339亿美元

自我保健总费用
220亿美元(64.9%)

从业者总费用
119亿美元(35.1%)

图27 2007年美国补充和替代医学的开销

余下的大部分，要么是从业者费用（119亿美元），要么是顺势疗法费用（29亿美元，尚不清楚这只是"药物"本身的数字，还是包括从业者费用在内的总成本）。无论如何，像美国这样爱打官司的社会，如此巨额的花费实属惊人。对于常规医学的从业者来说，通往从业执照之路漫长又关卡重重。任何获得批准的药物都经过了严格的审批程序以证明其药效、安全性，以及目的适用性。因此，从业者和使用的产品都有严格监管。无论是从业者还是药物和设备的销售商，任何人敢越雷池一步，必将受到严厉的处罚；任何人不按预期标准执行，都会招致法律的制裁，往往还会伴随着经济处罚。在常规医学中，制药公司在没有证据表明药物在合理的时间内有效的情况下，按照法律，就不得销售，哪怕只是哮喘药物。

　　对于大多数替代和补充医学来说，大多数国家都没有这样的检验。监管要么缺失，要么被包含在"专业"内。没有对比方说顺势疗法药物进行药效检验。这些专业的从业者为何不受制于这些基本的规则，让人无法理解。就算采用的是不同的规则，在根据某种货物或服务具有某种特性而收取费用的其他行业，如果该项商品或服务没有达到广告宣传的功能，也会受到法律的处罚。

　　事实是，这些疗法的提供者似乎相信它们都有效用，患者也如此认为。因此，替代和补充疗法实际上更像宗教而不是科学，这就在很大程度上解释了它们为何似乎享有法律豁免权，因为宗教本身在大多数国家也有着同样的法律特权。此外，临床试验中有一种众所周知的现象叫作"安慰剂效应"。盲法试验中的某些患者服用的是叫安慰剂的假药丸，他们常常也会体验到活性药物预期的良好效果（奇怪的是，有时还会体验到轻微的副作用）。这种效应往往十分可观，并且在很多方面是极为理想的——显然没有与药物相关的严重不良事件的风险。身体在进行自我治疗。因此，很显然，如果替代医学"从业者"和患者同样坚信某种疗法有效，它往往就会奏效。这说明它是一种可靠的做法吗？我觉得并非如此——我认为这些疗法无论是不是医学，都应该与其他任何产品一样，接受同样的效果检验。

此外，并不是说无效的产品就不会造成伤害——这取决于它如何改变了患者的治疗。比方说，如果顺势疗法被用来治疗软组织损伤等轻微的自限性病症，显然不大可能造成长期的伤害。如果（像某些顺势疗法的支持者倡议的那样）用它取代了治疗癌症、艾滋病或结核病的标准疗法，那么当患者放弃了某种更有效的治疗，病情显然会恶化。

正如已经讨论论过的那样，评估任何药物，无论是常规药物还是其他种类，黄金标准做法都是对照试验。这些做法广泛应用于评估常规医学，但也被用来测试诸如顺势疗法和针灸（对照组是假针灸组——针被插入，却是在"错误的"位置）等技术的补充或替代医学。

顺势疗法的基础是"以毒攻毒"。从业者取用能够引发恶心等症状的化合物，随后将其活性成分依次稀释到原物质一个分子都不剩下的程度。支持者声称构成顺势疗法的"强力作用"在某种程度上把具有药效的特性"印刻"在了水分子上。其效果一般被认为是顺势疗法开始时采用的药剂所引发症状的反面——因此，上面这个例子所得到的药物可以用来治疗恶心。这样的一种治疗要想奏效，需要大量改造物理学、化学和组织生 113

物学,而当前缺乏所有这些知识。就算我们承认自己关于这些学科的知识很不完善,希望能有临床试验的证据证明其药效也绝非不合情理。如果有令人信服的药效试验证据,那么显然就需要重新审视基础的科学正统来适应新的证据。因此,我们需要考察顺势疗法的临床试验证据。

实际上已经进行过一些顺势疗法的对照试验了。2005年,备受推崇的医学期刊《柳叶刀》(*The Lancet*)发表了一篇文章,分析了包含安慰剂在内的110个顺势疗法试验的结果。这些试验与110个类似的常规医学试验(在顺势疗法文献中称其为对抗疗法,意思是"与疾病不同")进行了比较。《柳叶刀》的文章得出结论说,在证实顺势疗法的相干效应的所有证据中,没有一种不能用安慰剂效应来解释。相反,常规试验能够表明,在同样的条件下,常规药物的效果远远超过安慰剂。因此,顺势疗法似乎在"替代"类别里坐稳了,因为其从业者鼓吹的正是如此:常规医学的一种替代品。在没有证据表明存在切实好处时,特别是在顺势疗法宣传可以应用于所有疾病,其中包括有致命危险的哮喘、结核病以及艾滋病的情况下,这看来是一种不负责任的观点。关于顺势疗法的这种观点得到了世界卫生组织等机构的支持,该组织近来发布了一个警告,称使用顺势疗法治疗诸如结核病和疟疾等疾病非常危险,该警告非常明确地说,如此可能会付出生命的代价。因此,从任何一个层面上来说,在我们审视顺势疗法的"科学"时,若以传统科学为尺度,它显然问题重重——其作用方式缺乏合乎逻辑的物理基础,药效方面也没有令人信服的试验证据。尽管缺乏证据,顺势疗法仍可以通过英国的国家医疗服务体系来获得,全世界也有数百万人相信它的

114

疗效,其中包括威尔士亲王①。

那么,为什么会有这么多患者使用这些治疗？大多数人对科学的理解都非常粗略,往往会把科学家和替代疗法从业者的说法看作是同样合理的选择。这种观点独独限于生物学——比方说,没有人愿意在工程或开飞机上使用"替代"方法;他们会严格遵守空气动力学定律,坚持采用受过培训的飞行员。我认为在很多乃至大多数情况下,人们只是感到绝望,想在二者身上都下重注。穷尽了常规治疗方案的患者往往会转向这些疗法,显然很容易被人利用。这些治疗的极端例子往往会要求患者去其他国家治病,那里对这种疗法的监管没有美国或欧盟等地那么严格。

患者经常还会采用不寻常的饮食疗法。其基本原理常常会把因与果混为一谈,如果那些疗法还谈得上有原理的话。这些饮食的基础逻辑大多是这样的:饮食中缺乏 X,患上某些种类癌症的风险就会增高(可能),因此,服用 X 就可以恢复平衡,从而治疗癌症。患者于是就开始服用比如维生素或矿物质补充剂。作为一项建议,这至少还是可以验证的——我们可以对有关的补充剂做试验,看看它是否会影响患者的治疗结果。抗癌饮食中的另一个常见的主题是将饮食中的某个具体成分作为众矢之的,例如动物脂肪,潜在的逻辑是很多常见的癌症都与饮食中的动物脂肪过量有关,因此停止摄入动物脂肪便可治疗癌症(不太可能)。只需在肺癌里把"动物脂肪"换成"吸烟"一词,就能说明这种做法徒劳无益——如果只靠戒烟就能治疗肺癌,就没有

---

① 指现任英国王储查尔斯。

几个人会死于此病了。遗憾的是，对于大多数肺癌可以预测到的严峻结果来说，戒烟的作用极其有限。同样，显然没有任何证据表明这种"减法"饮食能够影响癌症存活率。我在诊所患者身上观察到的另一个最近的例子是说吃糖很不好，因为这会给癌症"加油"。因为所有复合碳水化合物在被吸收之前都会在消化道内被分解为糖类，这个疗法成立的可能性微乎其微，尤其是考虑到肝脏和胰腺等器官都在密切调节着血液的含糖量。

尽管存在这些逻辑缺陷，并且缺乏证据，患者却往往会采用新的饮食来应对癌症的诊断结果，他们经常会放弃喜欢了数十年的食物，采用某种据称有"解毒"或"治疗"特性的饮食，或是添加补充剂来"提升"身体的防御机制。极端情况下，从业者和拥护者往往会以近乎宗教的热情来鼓吹这些方法。确实，坚守这些教条在很多方面都很像宗教仪式，认为拒绝接受和自我牺牲有可能会换来回报，提升幸福。和宗教仪式一样，无需药效的直接证据——相信它有用就足够了。此外，如果此方法未能奏效，则可以被解读为没有努力实践养生法，而不是它们本身缺乏疗效。

1990 年，我们一行三人（两个肿瘤科医生和一个精神科医生）走访了墨西哥蒂华纳市的热尔松中心。热尔松方案基于一套古怪的"解毒"饮食（严格素食，水果和蔬菜的带肉果汁，不加盐）以及坦白来说相当怪异的做法（定期用新鲜咖啡灌肠）。马克斯·热尔松博士研发出这种饮食法来治疗包括糖尿病（他治疗过阿尔伯特·史怀哲[①]）和结核病在内的各种病症。具有讽刺

---

① 阿尔伯特·史怀哲（1875—1965），德裔法籍通才，拥有神学、音乐、哲学及医学四个博士学位。他因为在中非西部加蓬创立了阿尔伯特·史怀哲医院而获得了 1952 年度的诺贝尔和平奖。

意味的是,他因为鼓吹治疗糖尿病的饮食疗法而被美国驱逐出境,当时对糖尿病患者采用的是高脂肪、低碳水化合物的饮食。后来证明,高纤维、低脂肪的"热尔松"饮食法实际上是一种很好的糖尿病治疗法,但人们意识到这一点,已经是多年之后了。这的确证明了有必要以科学的方式来评估各种疗法,评估以后,便证明了低脂肪、高碳水化合物饮食法对治疗糖尿病的价值。然而,热尔松在被美国驱逐出境后继续鼓吹治疗一系列其他疾病的疗法,其中包括癌症、心脏病和关节炎。1947年和1959年,美国国家癌症研究所进行了两次调查,评估热尔松养生法是否对癌症结果有任何影响,两次的结论都说它没有令人信服的疗效证据。1990年,我们自己在审阅了由该中心挑选的病例之后,也得出了同样的结论,发表在医学期刊《柳叶刀》上。该中心的患者无疑相信自己从中受益了,并且由于上文所列的原因,他们感觉能更好地掌控自己的命运,在某种意义上获得了附带的心理益处。然而,这也有负面的影响,有些患者在这些治疗中投入了大量精力和信仰,在病情恶化时难免会感到他们无论怎样努力都是徒劳。这本身往往就很痛苦了,有时还会迫使他们错误地认为,只要坚持到底,就一定会有所改善,因而更极端地坚持某种养生法。

热尔松疗法之类的饮食法还有另一个问题。尽管从某些方面来说,这种饮食法(至少要除去咖啡灌肠)可以被看作是健康的,它却有可能并不适合某些类型的癌症患者。例如,胰腺癌患者的体重往往会迅速降低。因此,遵循一种往往会导致健康个体降低体重的饮食法,对于体重降低也是迫在眉睫的一个问题的人来说,实际上是有害的。同样,如上文所述,很多患者会把常规医学和替代疗法"混搭"起来。化疗等疗法可能导致消化问题并促使体重降低。因此，极高纤维、总热量却相对较低的饮食在这种情况下显然并不理想。替代疗法的从业者当然会说，这里的问题在于常规疗法而不是替代疗法。如果这些疗法受制于适当的审查并证明有效，这句话本来也可接受。对于热尔松疗法来说，虽然已经应用了90年，有很多已经发表的临床病例报告和学术界的探讨述评，却仍然没有一个正式发表的临床试验。正如药物那样，我认为为这类疗法安排试验是倡导者的责任，就像制药公司必须证明其产品的药效才可以获得批准一样。或许的确有患者从"替代"饮食法中获益了，但目前还是缺乏证据。

与替代饮食法密切相关的是基于维生素和矿物质或混合草药（有时称作"食疗品"）的营养补充剂。与热尔松治疗师之类的群体鼓吹的彻底改变生活方式相比，这些疗法可能更易于进行常规临床评估。最简单的饮食补充是服用维生素或矿物质。维生素［vitamins，复合词"vital amines"（"维持生命所必需的胺类"）的派生词］是微量存在于食物之中的化学物质，对于机体维持正常功能必不可少。维生素C就是个很好的例子，它来自各种水果，特别是柑橘类。缺乏维生素C会导致古代水手的头号灾难——坏血病，这种疾病的症状包括伤口愈合障碍，组织脆弱、容易瘀伤流血，牙龈出血和牙齿脱落，即身体所谓的"结缔组织"无法正确地连接各部件。因此，维生素C显然对生命至关重要，但如果体内有足量的维生素C，服用更多是否有益？诺贝尔奖获得者莱纳斯·鲍林坚信，所谓的"超大剂量"维生素是有益的，他大力鼓吹用这种做法来治疗从普通的感冒到癌症等各种疾病（应该指出，他获得的是诺贝尔物理学奖，而不是医学

癌
症

奖）。现在我们有了一种很容易检验的假说——维生素C可以做成药片，像其他任何药物那样接受评估。在各种环境下充分评估之后，答案却是掷地有声的否定：超过正常水平的维生素C饮食补充无助于战胜癌症（或其他任何疾病）。尽管如此，缺乏药效的铁证还是无法阻止替代疗法从业者继续鼓吹该药剂的使用，随手上网一搜，就能看到它们的广告无处不在。

　　矿物质是更简单的物质，但对它们进行试验也非常困难。比方说，硒存在于蔬菜之中，还是身体组织的必要成分，参与维护上皮细胞膜，即机体各种管道和腺体的内膜细胞的完整性。正是这些细胞引发了常见的癌症，因此，硒看来是饮食补充的一种潜在的候选物。进一步研究表明，硒水平较低的人口患癌的风险较高。这激起了癌症患者服用硒补充剂的各种试验，一项著名的皮肤癌研究表明，补充额外的硒的患者患上另一种癌症——前列腺癌——的风险较低。问题在于，这并非此项试验的研究目的，但无论如何，这已经足够促使那些担心自己前列腺的男性大量摄入硒了。为了确认效果，美国举行了一次名为"SELECT"的大型试验，旨在调查两种补充剂——硒和维生素E。该试验招募了30 000名男性，以双盲的方式分配给他们一种或另一种补充剂、两种全有或两种皆无，但后来数据与安全监察委员会叫停了这个试验。到此时为止，研究人员跟踪这些男性的平均时间已有五年。该委员会发现，不但两种药剂均没有任何令人受益的迹象，更麻烦的是，硒有可能让患上前列腺癌的风险轻微上升，而出乎意料的是，维生素E也有可能让患上糖尿病的风险上升。

　　然而就连这也不见得能给这个主题盖棺定论。在北美，膳食中的硒含量相对较高,因此与膳食中的硒含量较低的欧洲(差异与蔬菜所生长的土壤的硒含量有关)相比,额外摄入硒可能没什么好处。此外,硒可以以纯粹的化学品形式,或是与有机化合物相联系的所谓"复合物"的形式来提供,后者更像是从食物中获得的形式。因此,我们可以确定的是,SELECT试验所使用的药片形式不能预防北美男性的前列腺癌。目前仍在用这两种药剂进行其他试验——例如,我们自己的小组正在研究硒和维生素E对早期膀胱癌(这也与饮食中缺乏这两种物质有关)男性和女性患者的作用,以观察补充剂是否可以防止癌症的复发。

我个人的观点是,在发达世界,大多数情况下多数膳食都提供了足量的大多数维生素和矿物质,特别是考虑到过度摄入热量的势头还在不断增长。在此背景下,补充剂的任何影响可能都是微小的,因为大多数膳食里的含量已经超出了人体真正需要的水平。这正是明确的试验证据如此难以获得的原因所在。就像生活中的很多事情一样,起初看起来相当简单的事情,越仔细端详,就会变得越复杂。这种不确定性当然为补充剂市场增添了活力——还有什么比服用额外的"天然"维生素和矿物质更安全的呢?如果那些穿白大褂的人(如今我们大多数时候当然不再这么穿着了)对这一点不确定,何不服用这些药剂以防万一呢?

草药又如何呢?与化学生成的粗糙药品相比,从更加"天然"的意义上来说,它们当然颇具吸引力。然而,这种逻辑在本质上存在缺陷——自然界里没有什么东西是天生"美好"的——随便看看关于野生动物的电视节目就可以确认这一点。在这个语境之下,"天然"一词实际上没有什么意义——语境决定一切。比方说，肉毒杆菌中毒是一种令人非常难受的消化道感染，有时还会致命，但肉毒杆菌毒素却被用于让人看起来更"美丽"，作为一种药品，显然也相对安全。因此，药品比其"天然"来源要安全得多。如果某种草药疗法有疗效，那当然是因为它是一种药物（或者更准确地说，是很多药物的合剂，活性各不相同，副作用也多种多样）。草药自古便有也毫无神奇之处（仿佛使用的长久时间给它戴上了光环似的）。长期使用的天然疗法的好例子包括金缕梅（含有大量水杨酸，也就是阿司匹林）、罂粟（吗啡和二乙酰吗啡的来源）以及毛地黄。毛地黄是古代药物来源的一个好例子。一种用毛地黄叶子调制的饮品名为"什罗普郡茶"，几百年来一直被用来治疗所谓的"水肿病"——下肢积水，伴以呼吸短促，如今称之为心脏衰竭。后来20世纪的科学从中分离出活性成分——洋地黄生物碱（以该植物命名的一族化合物），其中最常使用的是地高辛。这些药物至今仍是治疗心脏衰竭的主要成分。但据我所知，如今没有人再用什罗普郡茶来代替地高辛了。

那么，草药类的癌症药物怎么样？好吧，首先，很多癌症化疗药物实际上就是草药提取物——用来治疗血癌和淋巴癌的长春新碱就来自长春花。用来治疗包括乳腺癌、前列腺癌和肺癌在内的多种癌症的紫杉烷类药物则来自紫杉的树皮和树叶，诸如此类。因此，对草药性质的研究一直是我们某些最有效药物的一个卓有成效的主要来源。同样，这些药物的天然源头并不是良好的草药——例如，吃紫杉叶既困难（它们的质地非常粗糙），也有可能致命——有用的治疗效果和致死之间只有一步之隔。

草药得到检验的研究有很多例子。我特别感兴趣的一个是起初叫PC-SPES（是前列腺癌-*spes*的缩写，*spes*是拉丁文，意为"希望"）的合剂。这种合剂据称来自一种"古老的"草药疗法，是作为"前列腺保健品"上市销售的。大约20年前，前列腺癌主流试验中碰巧同时在服用PC-SPES的患者显然从这种草药疗法

中获益。抛开它的名字不谈，它的制造者并没有把它作为一种癌症疗法进行试验，而是当作一种食品补充剂获得批准。后来的实验室调查证实，PC-SPES的表现很像雌激素——严格地说，是一种植物雌激素。这让我们想起，雌激素类药物广泛用于前列腺癌的治疗，因而PC-SPES完全有可能具有抗前列腺癌的效果。对于患者服用这种合剂的详细研究证明，它对雄性激素水平以及前列腺癌标记物PSA会产生影响，后者与激素的作用基础相一致。临床和化学分析发表于《新英格兰医学杂志》（*New England Journal of Medicine*），那大概是世上首屈一指的医学杂志了。

这篇文章的发表促成了在晚期前列腺癌患者中比较PC-SPES和一种名为己烯雌酚的真正雌激素的一次试验。试验开始了，但因为PC-SPES受到己烯雌酚的微小污染而被提前叫停。制造商"植物实验室"随即被美国的监管当局查封，此项研究便再无可能完成了。这个故事有些令人费解的方面。PC-SPES生产多年都没有过任何负面调查，原发表于《新英格兰杂志》的文章的分析中也没有发现己烯雌酚的污染。此外，就已经完成的这项试验而言，它证明PC-SPES优于己烯雌酚，这个结果与某些评论者认为的因己烯雌酚污染所致的临床效果相左。

PC-SPES等药剂的问题在于，它们只是作为食品而获批的，

因此不像药物那样，必须经过种种严格评估。同样，制剂是草药提取物的合剂，让人不由得怀疑合剂中有多少成分是观察到的真实临床效果（其中包括深静脉血栓等已知的雌激素不良反应）所确实需要的。什罗普郡茶和地高辛的例子说明了潜在的研发¹²²路线。解开这个谜题当然要花多年时间和大量的医疗经费，还可能没有专利保护来让公司为这些成本筹集资金。因此，我们很可能永远都不会知道PC-SPES真正的活性成分是什么。此外，尽管该药剂看似有临床价值，却再也见不到了，虽说市面上有若干类似的药剂（名字各不相同，包括一种叫PC-HOPE的，让人直接联想到PC-SPES）并在患者中间广泛使用。这些PC-SPES的仿造品是否真的和原版一样，还是无从知晓。服用这些药剂的患者大多无人监督，关于剂量、不良反应等问题也没有成体系的文献资料。此外，因为这些都是草药合剂，即使各成分的分量都是一样的，也无法保证连续批次中实际活性成分的分量完全一样——侍弄过花园的人都知道，种在同一块土地上的植物每年都会发生变化。鉴于草药疗法的性质和当前的批准环境，我们很难看清前进的方向。因为"植物实验室"PC-SPES的遭遇，各公司不太可能在未来争相进行草药疗法的试验。同样，把一种草药合剂转变成常规药物的成本，以及有可能毫无专利的保护，也令人望而却步。制药业当然还会继续筛检有药用性质的草药，但后续研发的目的是取得单一的化学物质，而不是一种草药制剂。我怀疑这些制剂会永远停留在常规医学和替代医学从业者之间的灰色地带。这种情形令人遗憾，因为在槲寄生提取物一类的大量无效疗法中间，无疑会混杂着一些像PC-SPES一样的药剂，其活性有潜在的价值。

　　总之，在卫生经济中，补充和替代医学形成一项巨大而重要的经济活动。然而，大多数这类疗法的收益都缺乏直接的证据。此外，在某些情况下，有充分的证据表明它们**缺乏**收益。尽管如此，有很大比例的癌症患者仍然把这些疗法作为对其常规治疗的辅助（或在某些情况下取而代之）。在这些准医疗干预之外，还有另一个改变饮食结构、补充剂和草药疗法的领域，它们同样基本上没有什么证据基础。理解这些疗法的用途十分重要，因为它们可能会证伪癌症治疗试验的结果，也可能会干预常规治

疗的结果，无论是使其更好（这种情况极可能很少）还是更差。

索 引

（条目后的数字为原文页码，
见本书边码）

C

癌

症

癌症

索引

M

N

O

癌
症

S

索引

癌

症

索引

Nicholas James

CANCER

A Very Short Introduction

Contents

Acknowledgements

Writing even a small book such as this is a big undertaking. I'd like to acknowledge the help and support given by my wife Alison and by my family in giving me the time and space needed to produce this book. I'd also like to thank my parents for the massive contributions they made to supporting my education, often at great personal sacrifice.

List of illustrations

Genius

Chapter 1
The size of the cancer problem

Cancer is common, very common. In 2008, around 12.7 million people were diagnosed with cancer, of whom 7.9 million died, accounting for around 13% of all deaths. Although there is a perception that cancer is a disease of the aged population in the richer economies, around 70% of these deaths occurred in low- or middle-income countries. Cancer affects both genders, all races, rich and poor alike. The diagnosis is feared, as it is assumed (often correctly) to be a death sentence by those afflicted with it. Both the disease itself and its treatment are major causes of pain and distress. Treating cancer is a major burden on healthcare systems worldwide, and the disease is a significant cause of loss of productive capacity within the workforce due to premature death. This chapter will take an overview of the cancer problem, focusing on some of the more common cancers to illustrate how numbers vary across the world. Any illness affecting so many people will also have major economic impacts, so this chapter will also highlight some of the ways in which the economy and health services interact, themes that will be developed further in later chapters. Studying patterns in rates of cancer sheds very interesting light on the causes of cancer (covered more fully in Chapter 2). Some of the most striking links will be highlighted in this chapter as well.

Cancer care and cancer research are also important components of industrial activity. Half of all drugs in clinical trials are for cancer; the global market for all cancer drugs was estimated at $48 billion in 2008, up from $34.6 billion in 2006. Analysts expect growth from 2010 to 2015 to be above 10% annually. Every year, the pharmaceutical industry spends between $6.5 and $8 billion on research and development of cancer drugs. This spend dwarfs that from government and research charities on drug development, potentially meaning that new drugs are concentrated in areas with maximum commercial rather than public health impact. Pharmaceutical companies with successful cancer drugs are among the biggest corporations worldwide. Biotech companies without marketable products but with a promising 'pipeline' cancer drug can be worth billions of dollars simply because of the possibility that the drug may be licensed at some future date for treating cancer. At least 19 anticancer drugs exceeded $1 billion in sales in 2009, a major strain for health systems in even the richest economies charged with purchasing these drugs for their patients.

At the other end of the spectrum, around one-third of cancer patients have very limited access to effective treatments, rising to over half in the poorest countries. Moving forwards, with an ageing population and rising drug price trends, we may get to the situation when 'state-of-the-art' drug therapy will be available only to the richest strata in the richest economies. Alternatively, better prediction of response to therapy may allow individually targeted treatment choices, reducing costs from unnecessary or ineffective therapy. Unlike, say, cars or computers, which we expect to work every time we use them, most cancer drugs work on only a proportion of patients. For those with advanced disease, for whom the aim is palliation of symptoms or improvement in quality of life, this proportion may be much less than 50%, hence the majority of treatments may be pointless, or indeed worse than useless, as they may cause side effects with no benefit. Being able to identify patients who may benefit ahead of therapy would be very cost and clinically effective and this is therefore a major focus of current cancer research (see Chapters 4 and 5).

Cancer has also fascinated the world's academics and universities. In 1961, John F. Kennedy pledged to put a man on the moon by the end of the decade. Nine years later, Neil Armstrong and Buzz Aldrin walked on the moon. Ten years later, in 1971, Richard Nixon echoed this pledge by declaring a 'war' on cancer. Rather like the more recent 'war on terror', picking a fight with a multifaceted worldwide problem has been at best only partly successful. Nixon's initial pledge was around $100 million, which seemed like a bonanza at the time, but has turned out to barely scratch the surface. Since 1971, billions more research dollars have followed, but more than 30 years later cancer remains one of the largest causes of death worldwide, with around 1 in 3 developing the disease in developed economies and 1 in 5 in the West dying from it. Curing cancer is clearly harder than 'rocket science'.

Worldwide, huge amounts are spent on research into the causes and treatment of cancer. In 2009/10, the US National Cancer Institute spent $4.7 billion on cancer research; equivalent spend in Europe was around €1.4 billion. In the UK, the biggest spender is Cancer Research UK, one of the largest British charities, which in 2010 had an annual income from donations of more than £500 million, reflecting the importance attached to finding causes and cures for cancer among the wider population (the foremost recipients of public donations are, however, animals not people!). Despite this vast expenditure on research, we still do not really understand what causes a substantial proportion of cancers. Furthermore, despite the money spent on drugs and drug research, for the majority of patients cured of cancer, this is as a result of either surgery or radiotherapy, as described in Chapter 3. Chemotherapy and other newer treatments such as monoclonal antibodies or targeted 'small molecule' therapies, while growing in importance, still account for only a minority of cures but have a major role in palliation of advanced disease symptoms.

There are various ways of looking at the problem cancer poses. These range from the raw numbers – how many people diagnosed, how many people die – to the personal – what is your individual risk of getting a particular cancer? Population-based statistics can be presented in various ways, from rates for the whole population to rates adjusted by age to calculations on numbers of years of life lost. These latter statistics are often expressed as years lost before the age of 70 – the biblical 'three score years and ten' – thereby assuming that deaths after 70 (or sometimes 75) essentially represent death from old age. A further complication is that deaths from cancer vary enormously by income, race, and country of residence. For example, breast and prostate cancers are much more common in Europe and North America than in Japan and China. Migrants from these countries to the United States progressively alter their risk of these cancers towards that of white Americans but retain a lower overall risk. This tells us that the lower rates of breast and prostate cancer in the Far East are partly down to environment and partly down to racial differences or some linked aspect of the environment that is portable – diet, for example.

To try and explore these concepts further, I will present samples of the raw statistics using a range of methods. The question of which statistic is most useful depends on your point of view. For example, doctors working in public health, responsible for planning healthcare provision for a local population, will not be very interested in the rates of a given cancer in another country. Conversely, researchers looking at the effect of diet on risk of cancer may well want to focus on differences in disease rates between societies, as they may shed light on which lifestyle factors are important in the development of a given cancer. Fundraisers for cancer research will tend to focus on diseases affecting large numbers in the target donating population – breast cancer is the best example of this in Europe and North America, but more recently fundraising for prostate cancer has tapped into the same vein of public opinion.

The raw figures

As already mentioned, around 13%, or 1 in 7, of all deaths worldwide are due to cancer. This rises to around 1 in 3–4 in the developed world, where risk of premature death from infections, malnutrition, or violence is comparatively much lower. Figure 1 shows the numbers diagnosed with, and Figures 2 and 3 those dying from, cancer in different parts of the world. It is clear that there are large variations by region, with cancers common in one part of the world not featuring in the list of common cancers in another. There are too many differences to cover every one in detail. I will therefore highlight a few to illustrate why and how these differences arise.

Lung cancer

Worldwide, lung cancer is the largest cause of cancer death, with 17% of all cancer deaths, amounting to 1.2 million people, due to this type. It is a highly lethal disease, with fewer than 1 in 10 diagnosed surviving 5 years in most countries. Even in the United States, which has the best treatment results, fewer than 1 in 5 survive long term. Furthermore, the worldwide death rate is rising rapidly, having doubled between 1975 and 2002. Figure 1 shows the rates of diagnosis for different cancers around the world and clearly shows that lung cancer is among the major killers in all parts of the globe. There is a well-known, strong link between smoking and lung cancer. Differences in the rates of lung cancer not surprisingly therefore vary with rates of smoking. Mostly, lung cancer is diagnosed relatively late in life, reflecting consumption of large numbers of cigarettes over half a century in most cases (younger people who have had less exposure obviously can suffer from the disease, but these cases are relatively less common). It therefore follows that the rates of lung cancer and the trend in the rates (rising or falling) reflect smoking habits over the previous half century. If we know the trends in rates of smoking, we can predict the future trends in lung cancer rates for a population.

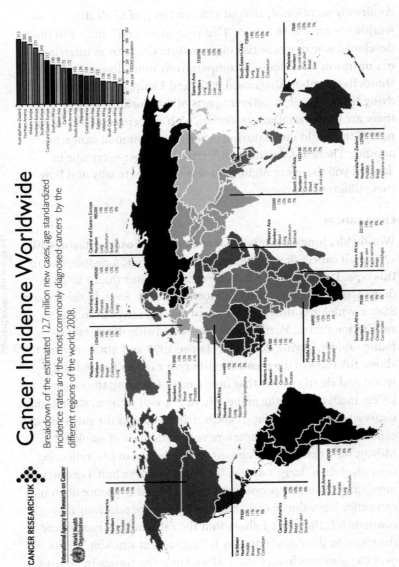

Cancer Incidence Worldwide

Breakdown of the estimated 12.7 million new cases, age standardized incidence rates and the most commonly diagnosed cancers by the different regions of the world, 2008.

CANCER RESEARCH UK

International Agency for Research on Cancer

World Health Organization

Northern America
Numbers 1603900
Lung 15%
Prostate 13%
Breast 11%
Colorectum 9%

Caribbean
Numbers 79300
Prostate 20%
Breast 11%
Lung 11%
Colorectum 9%

Central America
Numbers 176600
Prostate 12%
Breast 10%
Cervix uteri 8%
Lung 6%

South America
Numbers 650300
Breast 14%
Prostate 13%
Lung 8%
Colorectum 7%

Northern Africa
Numbers 164400
Breast 17%
Bladder 7%
Liver 7%
Non-Hodgkin lymphoma 6%

Western Africa
Numbers 184100
Breast 16%
Cervix uteri 16%
Liver 12%
Prostate 7%

Middle Africa
Numbers 66900
Breast 16%
Cervix uteri 12%
Liver 12%
Prostate 7%

Southern Africa
Numbers 79200
Breast 11%
Prostate 10%
Lung 8%
Cervix uteri 8%

Eastern Africa
Numbers 221100
Cervix uteri 14%
Breast 13%
Kaposi sarcoma 8%
Oesophagus 7%

Western Europe
Numbers 1094300
Prostate 16%
Breast 14%
Lung 7%
Colorectum 13%

Southern Europe
Numbers 713900
Colorectum 14%
Breast 13%
Lung 12%
Prostate 7%

Northern Europe
Numbers 495500
Prostate 16%
Breast 15%
Lung 12%
Colorectum 12%

Central and Eastern Europe
Numbers 988200
Lung 14%
Colorectum 13%
Breast 12%
Stomach 8%

Western Asia
Numbers 223300
Breast 15%
Lung 12%
Colorectum 8%
Stomach 7%

South Central Asia
Numbers 1431100
Cervix uteri 12%
Breast 12%
Lung 8%
Lip, oral cavity 7%

Eastern Asia
Numbers 3720700
Lung 17%
Stomach 16%
Breast 13%
Liver 12%
Colorectum 10%

South-Eastern Asia
Numbers 725600
Lung 14%
Breast 15%
Liver 10%
Colorectum 10%

Melanesia
Numbers 7000
Lung 12%
Lip, oral cavity 12%
Cervix uteri 10%
Liver 7%

Australia/New Zealand
Numbers 127000
Prostate 17%
Breast 12%
Colorectum 12%
Lung 9%
Melanoma of skin 8%

Australia/New Zealand 313
Northern America 300
Western Europe 288
Northern Europe 271
Southern Europe 245
Central and Eastern Europe 190
Eastern Asia 188
Caribbean 173
South America 172
South-Eastern Asia 140
Melanesia 139
Central America 134
Western Africa 134
Eastern Africa 123
Western Asia 113
South Central Asia 108
Northern Africa 105
Middle Africa 103
Middle Africa 92

rate per 100,000 population

1. Worldwide cancer incidence

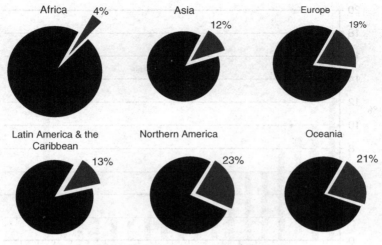

2. Proportions of people dying of cancer by continent

In Western Europe and North America, rates of smoking in men are declining and with them rates of lung cancer (and other smoking-related diseases). In contrast, in large tracts of the developing world, rates of smoking are increasing rapidly as countries industrialize. The effect this is likely to have on cancer rates is illustrated by trends in Japan, where the rate of lung cancer between 1960 and 1980 more than doubled as the effects of Japan's industrialization took their toll. Similar changes are now being observed in countries like China. There are various reasons for this: the habit still has an aura of 'coolness' in these countries very different from the increasing pariah status of smokers in the West. There are generally lower levels of awareness of the health issues attached to smoking, and the restrictions on tobacco promotion increasingly seen in Europe and North America are not present. Indeed, officials in one recession-hit Chinese province recently decreed that all adults had to smoke the local cigarettes in order to boost both the local growers and tax revenues. Looking forwards, therefore, we can see that just as lung cancer declines as

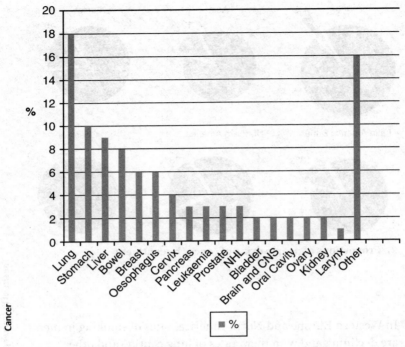

3. Causes of death from cancer worldwide

a problem in the 'developed' world, the newly industrializing economies will face an increasing burden of smoking-related cancers (and other problems such as heart disease) unless there is rapid adoption of the sorts of smoking-prevention strategies now the norm in Western Europe and North America. At present, this seems unlikely, and thus the industrializing world is likely to acquire one of the less desirable trappings of the developed world.

Breast cancer

In terms of new cases, breast cancer is the commonest cancer in women, accounting for 21% of female cancer cases and 14% of

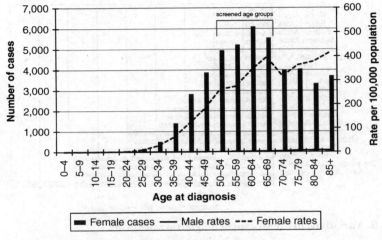

4. **Breast cancer diagnosis and death rates in the UK, 2005**

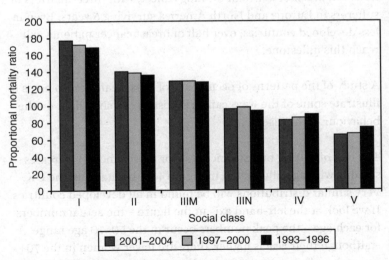

5. **Breast cancer diagnosis rates and social class**

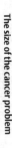

9

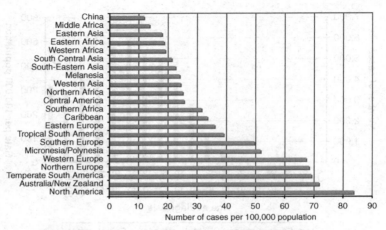

6. **Variations in breast cancer diagnosis worldwide**

female cancer deaths worldwide. The overall survival rate is, however, much better than for lung cancer, with three-quarters of sufferers in Europe and North America surviving 5 years. Even in less developed countries, over half of breast cancer patients will reach this milestone.

A study of the patterns of occurrence of breast cancer also helps to illustrate some of the ways cancer statistics can shed light on the behaviour of the disease.

The risk of getting breast cancer (as for most cancers) increases steadily with age, illustrated in Figure 4 with data from the UK. Very similar distributions will be found in all developed countries. If we look at the left-hand axis in the figure – the actual numbers for each age – the peak numbers occur in the 50–70 age range – although their risk is higher, there are fewer women in the 70+ age groups due to deaths from other causes. As can also be seen, few women aged under 40 are diagnosed with the disease, although fundraisers often use women from this age group in their promotional materials. The second figure, Figure 5, looks at the distribution of cases from another angle, that of social class. This demonstrates that wealthier, better-educated women are at significantly higher risk than the less well off. Middle-aged educated women are often formidable campaigners, having both the time and education to lobby effectively. As we shall see later in the book, neither cancer research nor treatment access are arranged purely on the basis of need but are often substantially influenced by lobby-group pressure on behalf of particular groups.

The figures on worldwide risk of breast cancer again show some striking trends. Looking at Figure 6, there is a clear suggestion that breast cancer is in some way associated with affluence – richer countries have higher rates than poorer ones. For the smoking/cancer link, there is a pretty clear relationship between consumption and risk. It is harder to see why higher average income should increase the risk of an illness – this is the reverse of most public health trends. So why should this be? One factor is the age structure of the population. As seen in Figure 4, risk of cancer increases with age. Hence a woman in a poor country with a low life expectancy may simply not live long enough to get breast cancer, having already died of another disease earlier in life. This does not account for the large range of risk seen, however. There are various theories about the observed underlying difference, and the most likely explanation relates to the effect of hormones on the breast tissue. For example, there are clear effects on cancer risk relating to age of first pregnancy and numbers of pregnancies. Late onset of puberty, early first pregnancy, and more frequent pregnancies are factors that appear to protect against breast cancer. In the West, puberty occurs earlier than in the past due to better nutrition and higher-protein diets, whereas pregnancy occurs later due to effective contraception, the increasing independence of women, and better education. In poorer countries, puberty occurs later and women have less control over their fertility. Whilst this situation of course brings all sorts of potential problems, it does appear to protect against breast cancer. Breast-feeding, which affects hormone levels post-delivery, also appears to protect against breast cancer, and being more prevalent among the better educated in the West may be predicted to skew the trend the other way. Fertility rates tend to drop and age at first pregnancy tends to rise as both national and personal income increases, so it may be expected that, as with lung cancer, increasing development will result in an increase in cases of breast cancer worldwide.

Clearly, the breast is an organ that changes throughout life in response to changes in hormone levels (arising from puberty, pregnancy, breast-feeding, menopause, or drug therapies such as oral contraception and hormone replacement therapy). It follows from the above observations that medical treatments that affect hormone levels may alter the risk of developing breast cancer. Hormone replacement therapy (HRT) is widely used for menopausal symptoms. It was hoped that, in addition to helping ameliorate symptoms such as hot flushes and loss of libido, HRT would prevent diseases that tend to occur with increasing frequency after the menopause such as heart disease and bone loss (osteoporosis) with consequent risk of fracture. While HRT is indeed effective in some of these aims, it also appears to increase risk of breast cancer with prolonged use. A similar effect is seen with the oral contraceptive pill, which again works by altering the normal hormone environment. These, then, are confusing effects: some hormone changes (those associated with pregnancy and breast-feeding) protect against breast cancer, while other changes (oral contraception and HRT) increase risk. Against this background, much laboratory research is focused on the role that hormones play in the causation of breast cancer and on the development of drugs that interfere with hormone pathways and thereby treat breast cancer. One of these drugs, tamoxifen, which acts mainly by blocking the effects of the hormone oestrogen, can be regarded as one of the most effective drugs of all time, having saved the lives of probably millions of women and helped prolong life for many more in the 25 or so years since it came into clinical use (see Chapter 3).

Finally, there is a perception, promoted to a degree by groups campaigning for better treatment and research, that breast cancer is a disease of young women. In general, as we have already seen, this is inaccurate. However, studies of patterns of risk of breast cancer revealed that some families appear to be at very high risk of breast cancer, with mothers, sisters, aunts all affected at an early age, often with disease in both breasts or associated with cancer of the ovaries, or of the prostate in the male relatives. These families were obvious candidates for in-depth study and, given the very obvious risks to the families involved, sufferers were often very receptive to participation in research. Studies of the patterns of inheritance in such cases suggested that the risk of breast cancer was passed on from mother to child with a 50:50 risk, and suggested at least two common inherited forms of the disease plus a number of less common versions. This is an area of research covered in more detail in Chapter 2.

Liver cancer

Liver cancer is one of the commonest cancers worldwide but with a very different pattern of distribution to lung and breast cancer. It is of particular interest as a freely available vaccination (against hepatitis B) can effectively prevent development of the cancer. Overall, it is the sixth most common cancer in terms of new cases, but the third most common cause of cancer death, reflecting the highly aggressive nature of the disease. There are a number of key features to the pattern of cases of liver cancer that merit more detailed examination. It is between 5 and 7 times more common in parts of China and Africa than in Europe and North America. The disease is almost always lethal, partly because it occurs in parts of the world with less developed healthcare, but mostly because it arises as a result of serious damage to the liver by the hepatitis B virus.

Liver cancer is linked to chronic liver damage, and in Europe and North America this is generally caused by alcohol abuse. In the parts of the world where the cancer is more common, the more important factor is infection with the hepatitis B virus (HBV), first described in 1965 by Dr Baruch Blumberg, who received the Nobel Prize for his work. Epidemiological studies established the link between hepatitis and liver cancer some years ago. Subsequent work showed that the molecular biology of the virus was consistent with it having a direct causative role rather than this being a chance association. With the linkage between virus and cancer established, the possibility of a vaccine against a common cancer became a reality. Pleasingly for all concerned, HBV vaccination has been a great success, with benefits appearing in the highest-risk populations very rapidly.

Cancers of the gut

Gut cancers commonly occur either in the top end (stomach and oesophagus) or the bottom end (colon and rectum), with cancers of the middle bit (the small bowel) being comparatively rare. There are some interesting trends in the patterns of gut cancers which I will run through, starting at the top with stomach cancer.

Overall, almost a million people are diagnosed with stomach cancer each year with around two-thirds of those afflicted dying from the disease – at least 650,000. Stomach cancer has been steadily falling in incidence in the West over the last 50 years, as illustrated in Figure 7, moving from being a relatively common cancer to now being quite rare. In other parts of the world, incidence has also begun to fall but more recently. Various reasons have been proposed for this, ranging from the rise of cheap refrigerators to medical treatments for stomach ulceration, but at present the reasons for the changes are not fully understood.

Cancers of the large bowel also show large variations between populations. Broadly speaking, bowel cancer is common in Europe and North America, less common in the Far East and uncommon in Africa. It is thus predominantly a disease of the developed world. Altogether, around a million people are diagnosed with the disease each year, and around half of these

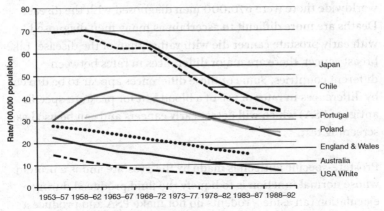

7. Rates of stomach cancer over time

patients will die from the disease. Death rates are now declining in North America and Europe due to improved awareness, early diagnosis, and better treatment. Studies of migrants suggest that the differences are environmental rather than racial – migrants from low-risk to high-risk countries rapidly take on the risk pattern of their new homeland. In addition, countries with an increasingly Westernized diet such as Japan are seeing a rise in the incidence of the disease. The prime candidate for this effect is therefore diet – differences in the environment of the lining of the lower bowel clearly arise from differences in what goes in at the top end! There thus appears to be some sort of reciprocal effect – changes in diet over the last 50 years have made stomach cancer increasingly rare but have led to an increased risk of cancer at the other end of the bowel. Studying these sorts of changes provides important clues to the origins of cancers and also can point the way to prevention strategies.

Prostate cancer

Prostate cancer is an interesting disease. In Europe and North America, it is the most frequently diagnosed cancer in men and one of the leading causes of cancer death in men. In 2007, worldwide there were 670,000 men diagnosed with the disease. Deaths are more difficult to ascertain as many men diagnosed with early prostate cancer die with rather than of the disease. Like breast cancer, there are major differences in rates between different countries. Some of these differences appear to be driven by differences in rates of use of a blood test for prostate-specific antigen (PSA) which will detect early cancers and can be used as a screening test.

Prostate-specific antigen is made by the prostate and is a protein whose normal function is to liquefy the fluid produced during ejaculation (an aside – rodents do not make PSA and produce a solid semen plug during intercourse, yet mice are widely used in prostate cancer research). PSA is found in small quantities in the blood in men without cancer. In the presence of a prostate cancer (but also in other diseases affecting the prostate), larger amounts are liberated into the bloodstream, enabling the measurement of PSA to be used as both an early diagnostic and monitoring test for prostate cancer. Since the early 1990s, the test has been increasingly widely available and used both for screening for undiagnosed cancer and as a tool for monitoring the response of the cancer to treatment. In the USA, the test has been widely available from a range of sources and is actively promoted to the public by the makers of test kits – knowledge of your PSA level has become something men need to be aware of in the same way that cholesterol used to be. In the UK, until recently, government policy discouraged 'opportunistic' PSA testing, and there was no systematic screening programme on the grounds that there was no evidence that early diagnosis of prostate cancer reduced death rates from the disease. Recent data from screening trials suggest that PSA testing may reduce deaths from prostate cancer, but that around 40 men need to be treated for PSA-test-detected cancer in order to save 1 life. Whether this level of benefit will result in screening programmes being set up remains to be seen. It should be noted that this is similar to the level of benefit from breast cancer screening. Although widely applied, the benefits of screening are therefore not nearly as clear cut as may be imagined from the very widespread application of breast cancer screening across the Western world. For the time being, PSA testing is variable across the world and largely consumer driven.

If we start by looking at diagnosis and death rates from prostate cancer, some very obvious differences are seen (Figure 8). Men living in Europe and North America have a strikingly higher death rate than men living in Indo-China, where the disease is relatively rare, as it is also in most of Africa. Within Europe and North America, there are further interesting variations, with increasing risk of death with increasing distance from the Equator, an effect best seen in the white populations of the United States and Australia where the ethnicity of the white population is fairly uniform. If we look at ethnic effects, there are also striking variations, with men of African origin having roughly double the risk of prostate cancer death than white men. In contrast, men of Indo-Chinese descent retain the lower risk of their regions of origin, similar to the effect seen with women and breast cancer.

How can we explain this? The best evidence suggests that the differences between the white and Asian populations are driven by differences in diet plus a difference in racial sensitivity to whatever causes prostate cancer (which is largely unknown). The variation with latitude is much harder to explain by diet and clearly is not explained by race, as it can be observed in Europe, North America, and Australia. The best explanation seems to be exposure to sunlight, with sun exposure being protective. This is a very surprising conclusion, given the widespread public health campaigns aimed at reducing people's exposure to the sun. How may sun exposure affect the risk of cancer in an internal organ about as protected from the sun as it is possible to be? The answer appears to be vitamin D. Lack of vitamin D leads to rickets and conjures up images of Victorian workhouses and deformed children, but the 21st-century version of the disease may be an increased risk of cancer, as summarized in the box.

17

Vitamin D, sunlight, and cancer

Vitamin D is closely involved in the growth and development of a whole range of tissues including glandular structures like the prostate and breast. Vitamin D metabolism is complex, but a key step occurs in the skin and requires sunlight. Lack of exposure to sunlight over prolonged periods may thus lead to a shortage of 'active' vitamin D – not enough to cause rickets, but enough to shade the odds of getting prostate cancer. This may also explain why men of African origin, who often have the darkest skins, may be at the highest risk of prostate cancer if living in temperate latitudes. If this hypothesis were true, it could be predicted that white people with the highest sun exposure in a population would have a lower risk of prostate cancer. A good index of sun exposure is skin cancer, and studies have been carried out of prostate cancer risk in those with skin cancer. As predicted, the risk of prostate cancer is reduced in those with the highest levels of sun exposure as evidenced by solar skin damage and skin cancer. What is more, with sun exposure, reduction in an individual's risk of getting prostate cancer is substantial – one study estimates this may be as much as 40%. Even in those developing prostate cancer, sun exposure appears to delay diagnosis significantly – around 5 years, from an average age of 67 years for the least sun-exposed to 72 for the most sun-exposed. The central message thus appears to be very consistent – one of the biggest killers of the male population could be prevented by more sunbathing – yet public health policy advises against it!

If this effect is present with prostate cancer, clearly mediated by circulating factors generated in the skin, could it be seen with other cancers as well? The answer appears to be 'yes', and the effect size seems to be similar for pretty much all cancers of internal organs. The only cancers that are increased by sun exposure are those of the skin (specifically melanoma), which

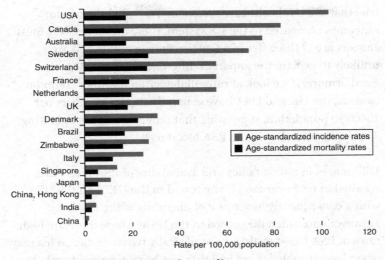

8. Prostate cancer incidence and mortality

actually kill relatively few people. The study of prostate cancer death rates thus sheds all sorts of interesting light on the causation of common cancers, and has thrown up a very surprising connection that fundamentally challenges current standard public health advice. In the opinion of the author, the accepted wisdom on sun exposure is overdue for radical revision.

There is a second striking set of differences in the diagnosis and death rates. If we compare, say, the UK and the USA, we see very similar death rates but very different diagnosis rates per 100,000 population, with more than twice as many cases diagnosed per death from prostate cancer in the USA as in the UK. Looked at another way, a far lower percentage of men with prostate cancer die from the disease in the USA than in the UK.

There are a number of possible explanations – prostate cancer may truly be more common in the USA, and the US healthcare system twice as good at treating it as the UK system. Whilst it is

19

true that the UK healthcare system delivers slightly inferior outcomes compared to the US system, these differences for most cancers are of the order of a few percentage points and are unlikely to explain the apparent difference in cure rates. Furthermore, if we look at rates of detection for other common cancers, the UK and USA have generally similar numbers per 100,000 population, suggesting that other factors are operating. The explanation lies in the PSA blood test.

Differences in public policy and availability of PSA tests have resulted in far fewer men being tested in the UK than the USA, with a consequently lower rate of diagnosis of the disease. However, most men diagnosed in the USA, where there are high rates of PSA blood testing, have clinically trivial disease. This may never have troubled them had they not been diagnosed with it, suggesting the large difference in incidence is largely driven by higher rates of diagnosis of low-grade, relatively non-lethal disease in the USA compared to the UK. Both sides of the Atlantic, a smaller number of men are diagnosed and eventually die from more aggressive forms of the disease. Since the late 1990s, death rates have been falling, but whether this is down to screening directly or to other factors is hotly debated.

Politics of cancer care

There are clearly many angles to the politics of cancer care, and these are linked closely to the economics of the disease. For the purposes of this chapter, I will focus on the differences in cases diagnosed and death rates and how they drive the politics of the disease, using breast and prostate cancer to illustrate gender differences and breast and lung cancer to illustrate social class effects.

In many ways, prostate cancer is the male counterpart of breast cancer. The similarities extend to a number of levels: both organs have a role in sexuality and reproduction; both change during life in response to hormone levels; both cancers can be treated by changes in the hormone environment; and treatments for the cancers arising in the respective organs cause profound changes in sexual function. Politically, the powerful sexual and emotional imagery of the breast has been used to great effect to channel research and treatment funds into breast cancer for many decades. This has resulted in steady and progressive improvement in outcomes for women with breast cancer, reflected both in improved survival and reduced damage from successful treatment. For example, women are increasingly offered less mutilating surgery or breast reconstructions rather than radical mastectomy. On the drug funding issue, women have again been very effective at campaigning for new treatments – witness the rapid uptake of trastuzumab (better known as Herceptin) across the European and North American healthcare systems.

Until recently, despite the biological parallels, there was no analogous movement to support men with prostate cancer or campaigning to improve treatments and outcomes. As recently as 1995, for example, spending on prostate cancer research in the UK was only one-tenth that on breast cancer. In the last 10 years, this has changed, partly driven by the PSA test. This shifted the spectrum of prostate cancer substantially to the 'left', with a decrease in late cases and increase in early cases for which the treatment options are more varied and the possibility exists for cure or prolonged survival with the disease. This historical lack of public health and research interest is particularly surprising given the general concentration of political and economic power in the hands of men of middle age and above – those most at risk of the disease and with very little risk of breast cancer (though men can get it). The difference appears to be rooted in the differing psychologies of men and women – it's fine for women to talk about breast cancer, and women are not seen as diminished but often rather strengthened by it – witness Kylie Minogue's recent world tour. On the other hand, it has previously been very difficult for men to talk about the disease, particularly when treatments carry 'unmacho' risks such as impotence and incontinence, quite apart from the fundamentally embarrassing route needed for diagnosis (via the rectum). Coupled with most men's general 'ostrich' approach to all matters related to health, the result has been a price paid by men living shorter, less healthy lives than women.

More recently, however, there has been a shift in public and economic policies, with more money spent on treatment for men and research into the disease. This has been driven no doubt in part by the pharmaceutical industry's belated realization that there is a lot of money to be made from one of the biggest male cancer killers in the West. There has also been a change in that major public figures such as Colin Powell, Roger Moore, and Rudolph Giuliani have been prepared to talk about their treatment for the disease.

Finally, the issue of smoking and public policy is worth mentioning in the context of the politics of cancer care, as this has varied widely across the world and over the decades. Not too long ago, tobacco companies actually ran adverts with the strap-line that a particular cigarette was the preferred brand for doctors. The linkage of smoking to increased risk of various cancers has been one of the triumphs of epidemiological research, and has resulted in massive reductions in the rates of smoking and diseases linked to it in the developed world. A range of measures has driven this, from legal (smoking bans) through educational (advertising and sponsorship bans, health warnings) through to fiscal (tax the stuff, which has the additional benefit of paying for the healthcare needed to pick up the consequences for smokers). In the developing world, things are different, however: smoking is still seen as 'cool', underpinned by advertising and marketing to young people, rather than the pariah activity banished to chilly doorways it has increasingly become in Europe and North America. Furthermore, the money brought in to developing countries by the big multinational tobacco companies carries with it much political clout, and this can used to tone down the public health assault on the habit that has occurred in the West. Coupled with the young age structures of developing countries, an epidemic of developing world smoking-related cancers – lung, bladder, throat, mouth – can be anticipated in the coming years. In countries like China which are rapidly modernizing and improving living standards and life expectancy, this can be expected to result in particularly large increases in these cancers.

Chapter 2
How does cancer develop?

In order to understand how cancer develops, it is necessary to include a little background on basic cell biology. The cell is the basic building block that makes up all living things. The human body, in common with all animals from the smallest such as yeast to the largest blue whale, is composed of cells. Some animals – yeast, for example – are made of single cells; others, ourselves included, are made of many different sorts of cells – blood, bone, brain, kidney, and so on. All cells in an organism have their own carefully controlled life cycle. Cancer occurs when the control of this cycle goes wrong, leading to unregulated growth of a group of cells which can spread and damage other structures in the body. This chapter will focus on how cancer develops and also on some of the underlying biology needed to understand this. I will also illustrate how an understanding of the causes can be used to define treatment strategies.

The key component of the cell for understanding cancer is the nucleus, which holds the DNA that contains the genetic code. Figure 9 shows a diagram of a DNA molecule. Cancer is caused fundamentally by damage to the DNA leading to abnormal, unregulated growth of cells. Remarkably, although different cells may differ markedly in their appearance and function (for example, nerve cells, muscle cells, and blood cells), all the cells in a given organism share the same DNA code. DNA is clustered into long strands called chromosomes. There are 23 pairs in each human cell. Within each chromosome, the DNA is arranged in genes, each one coding for a single protein. We can think about genes and chromosomes as being like a library of books, with each of the 23 chromosomes an individual volume and each of the 21,000 genes a page of instructions in that volume. It is easy to see conceptually how damage to a page of instructions can lead to alterations in the properties of a cell. This chapter will run through how these different structures work and interact, and how they can go wrong to lead to the development of a cancer.

Everyone starts life as a single fertilized egg that develops first into a ball of identical cells and then, progressively, grows, organizes, and develops into a complete complex individual. The process by which cells develop from this initial group into highly specialized subtypes is one of the most incredibly complex processes in nature and yet is happening constantly all around us and within us. This clearly requires an intricate network of checks and balances. It requires that cells communicate with their neighbours to ensure that the right development path is followed at the right time. It requires that cells no longer required are deleted and eliminated with the minimum of disruption (a process called apoptosis, from the Greek word meaning 'a falling off of petals'). As organs develop, they must grow their own blood supplies and maintain them in response to damage. It requires that organ systems communicate with each other, for example nerves connecting with the muscles they control. Endocrine (hormone) glands are coordinated to produce their products in cycles (for example, the ovaries) or in response to stress (the adrenal glands). This is achieved by genes being switched on and off in a coordinated fashion as individual organ systems grow and develop. Once the growth process is complete and the animal is formed, tissues must be maintained, damage repaired, and general housekeeping kept ticking over – nutrients supplied and processed, waste products eliminated, and so on. The more one thinks about the

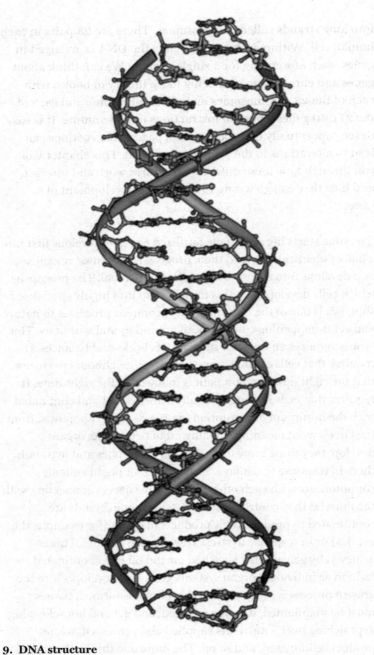

9. **DNA structure**

mind-blowing complexity of all these tasks, the remarkable thing is that the processes run so reliably for so many years in most people, and that cancer – essentially, unregulated cell division – does not occur more frequently than it does.

DNA structure and function

As already mentioned, the genetic code is stored in human cells in 23 pairs of chromosomes. Each chromosome comprises a very long molecule of DNA containing the genes, which are interspersed with spacer sequences. Each gene is flanked by regions of DNA that control when a particular gene is switched on or off. For example, the gene coding for the protein myosin, a key component of muscle cells, will be switched on where needed – in muscle – but off in other tissues where it is not required, such as nerve cells. The network of on and off switches is clearly critical to regulation of the behaviour of cells, and study of these controls is a major feature of cancer research – if the controls do not work, cells can grow in an unregulated fashion, as occurs in cancers.

To understand how cells carry out all these functions, it is necessary to understand a bit more about the structure of DNA and how the code embedded in the DNA molecule is translated into the end product that is the functioning organism. DNA is an abbreviation for deoxyribose nucleic acid. It had been known for some time before the famous discovery of its double helical structure by Crick and Watson in 1953 that DNA contained the genetic code. The DNA molecule (illustrated in Figure 9) is a long spine of two alternating building blocks – a sugar (called deoxyribose) and a phosphate group linked to four molecules named adenine, guanine, cytosine, and thymine (abbreviated to A, G, C, T) and referred to as bases. These bases are arranged along the spine of the DNA molecule and form two complementary pairs, A with T and C with G, that can bond to each other. The double helical nature of DNA results from one strand (the positive or sense strand) being matched by a complementary antisense strand with an A paired with every T, C with every G, and so on. The A–T and C–G bonds thus provide the 'glue' that maintains the double helical structure of the DNA strands. The complementary nature of the bond process means that if the two strands are pulled apart and each used as a template for two new strands, the result is two identical copies of the first DNA molecule.

This inherent property of DNA, whereby it can make identical copies of itself, is one of the fundamental properties of all life on Earth. The structure of DNA is very tightly conserved across the whole spectrum from the simplest to the most complex. The fidelity of the duplication process is also extremely high. The error rate is so low that it takes many generations to accumulate significant differences – the rate of genetic 'drift' – and is one of the bases for evolutionary biology. Coming back to the genetic books in the library: each time a cell divides, a complete set of the 23 pairs of volumes with their 21,000 genes ('pages' of information) must be 'typed' by the cell. From time to time, a comma, letter, or full stop will be mistyped. Mostly, as in a book, this will not alter the meaning, but sometimes, changes will be critical, with consequent alteration to how the daughter cell carrying the change (called a mutation) functions. Parenthetically, the number of small random differences can be tracked across the evolutionary tree to allow estimates of when a given pair of species diverged from each other.

Genes and control of gene expression

The fundamental unit that the DNA is organized around is the gene. A gene contains the code for a single protein. Proteins can have many functions ranging from structural, for example a protein called tubulin which makes the cell's internal 'skeleton', to functional, such as forming the parts of muscles that contract. This flow of information, whereby information in DNA is transcribed into a message (in RNA) and then into a single protein, is one of the central concepts of biology.

Proteins are the key building blocks of cells, responsible for all the key activities. Other components of cells, such as fats and sugars, are manufactured as a result of actions of proteins. Proteins clearly have to have a range of functions, therefore. These include: signalling both within and between cells; structure (a sort of microscopic scaffolding); and, very importantly, proteins called enzymes, which act on other biological molecules to bring about the formation of new molecules. This process can be destructive – for example, the enzymes in digestive secretions (and washing powders!) which break down food; or constructive – the enzymes involved in the manufacture of new molecules for the cell.

The production of a protein from a gene involves the transcription of the gene into a messenger ribose nucleic acid (mRNA) molecule within the nucleus of the cell. The RNA molecule has a structure like DNA but differs in key respects. Firstly, the deoxyribose sugar (the D in DNA) in the backbone is replaced by ribose (the R in RNA). Secondly, the molecule is single-stranded. And thirdly, the thymine (T) base is substituted by uracil (U), though the pairing remains the same.

In order to make RNA, the DNA double helix is temporarily 'unzipped' into two single strands. A complementary RNA molecule then assembles and is transported out of the nucleus into the cytoplasm and the DNA then zips itself back up again. This process, another key part of biology, is called transcription and is illustrated in Figure 10.

Once in the cytoplasm, this messenger RNA must be converted into protein, the second key part of the translation of the code embedded in the DNA into functional proteins. A second sort of RNA – called transfer RNA – provides the link between the messenger RNA and the building blocks of protein. Key to this translation process is the triplet code embedded in the DNA. Proteins, like DNA, are made up of chains of simpler molecules. The protein building blocks, called amino acids, can be linked

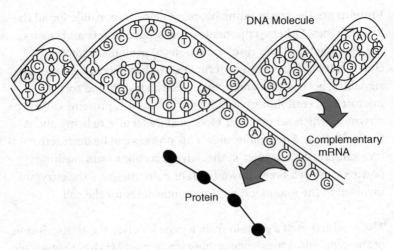

DNA Molecule

Complementary mRNA

Protein

10. Transcription

together to form effectively endless chains. The basic amino acid molecule has three key features – termed a carboxy terminus and an amino (hence the name) terminus, plus a variable side branch which gives each amino acid its distinct properties (illustrated as R in Figure 11).

Whilst in theory an infinite number of types of amino acids are possible, only 20 are found in living organisms. The DNA code is arranged in triplets called codons. There are 64 possible three-letter codes using A, T/U, C, and G. Each triplet has a specific meaning and can either refer to an amino acid or, in effect, form a punctuation mark. For example, within this coding system, AUG means 'start here' (termed a 'start codon'); UAG, UGA, and UAA mean 'stop here'; while the remainder are linked to specific amino acids – for example, cysteine is UGU or UGC. As there are 64 possible combinations in the triple code but only 20 amino acids, it follows that some amino acids have more than one triplet code. It can easily be seen, therefore, that a mutation which changes a single base can fundamentally alter the resultant protein. For example, a

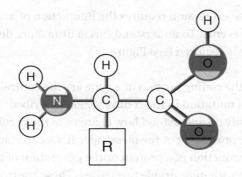

Amino acid (1)   Amino acid (2)

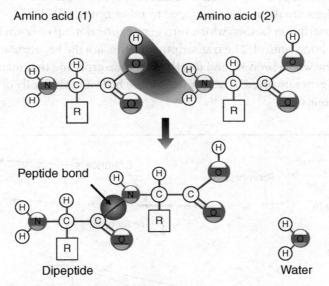

Peptide bond

Dipeptide   Water

11. Amino acids and protein structure

change from UGC (cysteine) to UGA (the stop signal) will shorten the resultant protein, with a possible major change in function.

As already mentioned, the core code of the gene is flanked by complex regulatory machinery (see Figure 12) to ensure genes are switched on and off at the correct times. It is this regulation of gene function that is often faulty in the cancer cell.

Regulation of gene expression requires the interaction of a complex series of events. To understand this, a little more detail on gene structure is required (see Figure 12).

On both sides of the coding portion of a gene are the control regions. As with a mutation in the coding region described already, it can easily be understood how changes to the regulation of the gene or the processing of the messenger RNA can result in over- or under-production of a protein or the generation of an abnormal protein with undesirable properties. These control regions are themselves regulated by other genes, called transcription factors, which turn gene expression up or down like a volume control. The transcription factors are the key regulators of the whole process, and it is therefore unsurprising that many of the genes involved in cancer turn out to be from this family of proteins.

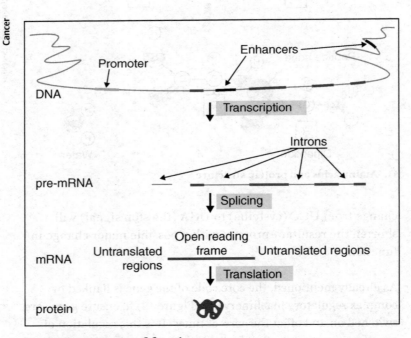

12. **Gene structure and function**

The hallmarks of cancer

Having covered the basics of the machinery, we can now turn to the ways in which the processes go wrong to produce a cancer. In 2000, two leading cell biologists, Douglas Hanahan and Robert Weinberg, published a seminal paper entitled 'The Hallmarks of Cancer' summarizing the changes that are both necessary and sufficient to produce a cancer. A cancer cell differs from normal cells in that it divides in an unregulated fashion. In addition, cancer cells have the ability to spread to and invade other parts of the body. Hanahan and Weinberg summarized the processes that must occur in the cell in order for it to be transformed from a normal, law-abiding member of cellular society into a dangerous outlaw. These changes, illustrated in Figure 13, are characterized as:

- self-sufficiency in positive growth signals;
- lack of response to inhibitory signals;
- failure to undergo 'programmed cell death' to eliminate faulty cells;
- evasion of destruction by the immune system;
- the ability to grow in and destructively invade other tissues;
- ability to sustain growth by generating new blood vessels.

The first two of these are reasonably self-explanatory and lead to unregulated growth. The third is less obvious and is linked to the development process. If all cells simply grew and divided, it would not be possible, for example, to form hollow tubular structures such as the gut or blood vessels. To do this, certain cells must be deleted from the growing organism as the needs of the growing structure dictate. This process, already mentioned, is called apoptosis, and is a key cellular function. Apoptosis is also a method that the organism uses to get rid of faulty or malfunctioning cells such as those nearing the end of their lifespan that need replacing. Cancer cells are by definition abnormal and thus should be self-deleting. Failure to undergo apoptosis is thus key to the transformation from an abnormal cell into one with limitless replicative potential. A further feature of apoptosis is that cells damaged by chemotherapy or radiotherapy

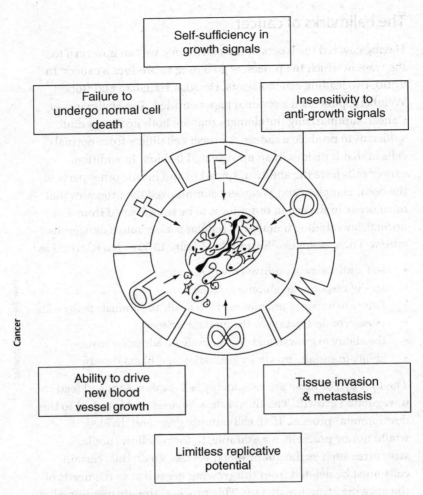

13. The hallmarks of cancer

are frequently not killed outright, but merely 'mortally wounded'.
The subsequent death of the cell is often by apoptosis, illustrating
that the evasion mechanism is not completely shut down, even in
the cancer cell. Increasing resistance to apoptosis is, however, one
way in which the cancer cell evades destruction by chemotherapy
or radiotherapy (see Chapter 3). Understanding apoptosis is

unsurprisingly therefore one of the major areas of cancer research.

Further distinguishing features of cancers are their ability to grow and to invade other tissues in the body while avoiding destruction themselves by the immune system. The immune system can be regarded as a sort of cellular police force that identifies intruders such as bacteria and eliminates them. As cancer cells are abnormal, the immune system should be able to identify and destroy them. Evasion of this process is therefore essential to the cancer. As already indicated, the growth and development of cells, tissues, and organs is very finely regulated to ensure the correct sort of cell grows in the correct place and time in the organism. One key aspect of cancer growth is the acquisition of the ability to grow in the wrong place, and this is a feature that distinguishes a malignant tumour from a benign one, which can grow but not spread or invade. It should be noted that benign tumours can still present severe consequences, for example an acoustic neuroma is a benign tumour of the auditory nerve that transmits signals from the inner ear to the brain. The tumour will progressively enlarge, causing deafness and balance problems, without ever spreading elsewhere.

The final hallmark of cancer is the ability to grow a new blood supply. Any collection of cells larger than around one-tenth of a millimetre across needs a blood supply. As the new tumour grows, it must therefore acquire the ability to stimulate blood vessel growth. The blood vessel growth of tumours is often haphazard and turns out to use genes not involved in the maintenance of normal blood vessels. The process is known as tumour angiogenesis, and because it differs from normal angiogenesis, it has become an important target for cancer drug development. If it is possible to knock out the blood supply of the cancer, further growth is prevented. One of the most successful of the new generation of targeted molecular therapies, bevacizumab (Avastin), works by targeting this process.

Carcinogenesis – how cancers start

As already indicated, cancer results when the changes required for the hallmarks of cancer have occurred. To understand how cancer develops, we now need to turn to how external factors bring about cancer – a process known as carcinogenesis. Fundamentally, cancer results from damage to DNA, leading to the changes described above and illustrated in Figure 13. All agents that damage DNA therefore are potential carcinogens – agents that cause cancer. The reverse is not true, however; not all agents that help cause cancer themselves directly damage DNA, though this always lies at the end of the process. Examples of cancer-causing substances that do not directly damage DNA include alcohol and the sex hormones involved in causing breast and prostate cancer. There are many sorts of carcinogens and many are well known – cigarette smoke and ionizing radiation, for example. Taking cigarette smoking, we know that typically it is necessary to smoke many cigarettes for many years for cancer to develop. This suggests that the process of carcinogenesis is slow and potentially has more than one step. From the discussion above, it would be predicted that mutations would be necessary in different sets of genes to cause the hallmark changes described by Hanahan and Weinberg. Such a chain of events was also postulated in the early 1990s and is now often referred to as the 'Vogelstein cascade', with each step in the chain representing a new mutation (Figure 14).

Dr Vogelstein's group studied inherited bowel cancer, a condition in which there are a number of recognized pre-cancerous (also called pre-malignant) steps that could be identified in patients. They collected tissues from patients and set about identifying which genes were abnormal in the various steps along the pathway from normal bowel lining to a clinically obvious cancer. It turned out to be possible to identify candidate genes that need to be damaged for each step of the cascade to occur. Subsequent work has demonstrated that similar cascades of events apply to all

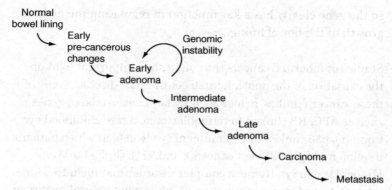

14. The Vogelstein cascade

tumour types, though the individual genes involved and the sequence of damage vary.

One fruitful way to identify genes has been to study families with so-called 'inherited' cancers. The term is a bit of a misnomer as the cancer is not inherited in the same way as, say, a diamond necklace, that is, as an intact, fully formed object. What is inherited is a greatly increased risk of developing a disease early, often in a very florid, aggressive form. One such disease is called adenomatous polyposis coli (APC). Patients with the disease develop multiple benign adenomas from an early age. In time, some of these progress to cancer, and without treatment death typically occurs in the early 40s from bowel cancer. Studies of patients with the disease showed that they had abnormalities in a particular gene, which was named APC. The identification of the APC gene in these patients led to further study of the function of the gene, which turns out to function as an 'off-switch'. If it is knocked out, an important check on cell growth is removed and adenomas form. As is often the way with inherited cancers, the much commoner, non-inherited cancers turned out to share similar abnormalities. Studies of non-inherited bowel cancer confirm that the APC gene is malfunctioning in around 80% of these sporadic cases, so the gene clearly has a key function in regulating the normal growth of the bowel lining.

Studies of inherited cancers thus often shed important light on the causation of the non-inherited counterpart disease. Study of these 'cancer families' helped identify key cancer-related genes such as APC, RB (linked to retinoblastoma, a rare childhood eye tumour), p53 (linked to Li-Fraumeni syndrome, in which patients develop multiple different cancers), and VHL (linked to von Hippel Lindau syndrome, a complex disorder that includes kidney cancer). In addition, examination of the varying natural history of the inherited disease helps us to understand what the normal function of these genes may be. All of the genes mentioned above are termed 'tumour-suppressor' genes, but this is a misnomer as this is not their primary role in the organism. As may be predicted from the APC gene, these genes are key regulators of the cell cycle (the first two aspects of the hallmarks mentioned above), and damage or deletion of function leads to uncontrolled growth. Examining the normal functions of these genes has shed important light on how the cell cycle is regulated. As lack of control of the cell cycle is a hallmark of cancer, many cancer treatments work by interfering with the cell cycle genes that are misfiring in the cancer cell. In addition, a new generation of cancer drugs, the targeted molecular therapies, is currently hitting the clinics and the news headlines (see Chapter 3). These drugs work by targeting specific molecules known to be misfiring in the cancer.

Not all inherited cancer genes are directly involved in the cell cycle, however. A good example is the VHL gene, originally identified in patients with von Hippel Lindau syndrome. Sufferers develop multiple abnormalities from an early age, including cysts in the nervous system, in particular the cerebellum (part of the brain involved in balance and coordination), spinal cord, and retina, together with kidney tumours both benign and malignant. The kidney tumours are typically bilateral, multiple, and occur from a young age. As for APC, the patient inherits one non-functioning gene; a single hit to the remaining gene leaves no functioning VHL protein in the cell. Given that renal tumours are relatively rare but are common in patients with VHL, this tells us that the chances of a given gene suffering one hit are relatively high, but suffering two hits takes much longer, hence sporadic tumours are single and have a much later age of onset.

Detailed study of the VHL gene has revealed that it is involved in sensing the oxygen levels in the cell. If oxygen is low, this leads to the production of signals to surrounding cells to start growing new blood vessels. In other words, it regulates angiogenesis, a key hallmark of cancer (see Figure 13). Further studies have shown that these changes are sufficient to drive the cancer cell in the test tube, and the replacement of the VHL gene in these models will reverse the cancerous characteristics of the cells. Furthermore, the kidney tumour type found in VHL patients, called renal cell carcinoma, is characteristically very rich in blood vessels, as may be predicted from the gene function. Study of sporadic (non-inherited) renal cell carcinomas has revealed that VHL is mutated in around 70% of cases, making the VHL/angiogenesis pathway an attractive target for therapy. Research into new VHL-based treatments for kidney cancer, a notoriously difficult cancer to treat once it has spread, has proved very fruitful, with six agents licensed since 2006 and several more pending for a disease for which only two agents had been licensed in the previous 25 years. All of these agents target aspects of the pathway identified by the genetic research summarized above.

Non-inherited cancer

While inherited cancers shed important light on the classes of genes involved in cancer, the majority of cases of cancer do not result from an obvious inherited predisposition. As we have seen in Chapter 1, the major causes of cancer death worldwide arise from tumours in the lung, stomach, liver, colon, and breast. Of these cancers, lung cancer is strongly linked to cigarette smoking, and liver cancer to infection with the hepatitis B virus, with a significant role for alcohol consumption. Cancers of the digestive tract are presumed to be linked to diet, but the precise causation is still poorly understood. Likewise, breast cancer (and prostate cancer in men) is clearly linked to both dietary and hormonal factors. How may these diverse influences act to produce the changes required to generate a cancer described above?

Lung cancer is the best understood example of how a carcinogen in the environment can interact to generate a cancer. The risk is clearly linked to amount of tobacco consumed – there is a dose effect – and the duration of consumption. Smokers who give up tobacco before getting cancer have a decreasing risk of developing the disease after stopping. In terms of a model like the Vogelstein cascade, smoking must be responsible for inducing the first steps of the cascade and continued smoking must also induce the subsequent steps. In older models of carcinogenesis, the initial step was often referred to as initiation and the subsequent steps as promotion of tumour growth, with a final step termed transformation. These terms still have value and in the laboratory, agents that convert non-malignant cell growths into cancerous ones are often referred to as transforming the cells. Analysis of tobacco smoke has revealed a host of agents that will result in transformation in cell culture systems. Detailed study of these smoke constituents has revealed the precise molecular mechanisms at work, down to the mode of interaction with the DNA double helix. One of the key culprits is called benzopyrene, and careful research has demonstrated it will bind to the DNA helix, damaging the structure. Figure 15 shows the benzopyrene molecule bound within a DNA double helix.

As mentioned above, there is clearly a need for DNA damage – an initiating event followed by a generally prolonged period of further damage accumulation, sometimes referred to as

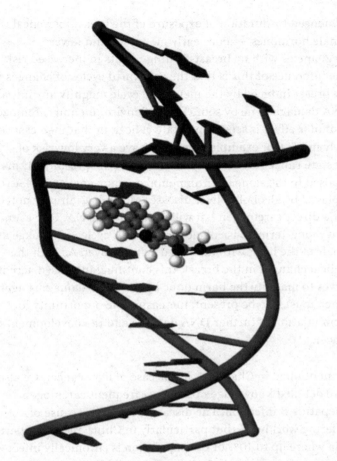

15. Benzopyrene bound within DNA

promotion – before a final transforming event turns the pre-cancerous lesion into a full-blown cancer. In the case of tobacco, the process appears to be driven by continuous exposure to tobacco smoke, which has direct DNA-damaging properties. For other diseases, in particular breast and prostate cancers, the role of promoter is taken by the individual's own hormones. As indicated in Chapter 1, risk of breast cancer is influenced by duration of exposure of the breast to cyclical female hormones – hence early menarche and fewer pregnancies with no breast-feeding results in increased risk. The inference of this is that the continued cycles of changes in the breast induced by the menstrual cycle magnify any initial DNA damage done by some form of environmental carcinogen. A similar effect is seen in prostate cancer, in that men castrated early in life (for example, eunuchs) have a very low risk of prostate cancer compared to their peers who presumably are exposed to the same environmental carcinogens. A similar role is played by alcohol in liver disease. Alcohol, as already noted, is not a direct carcinogen – it will not damage DNA. However, heavy long-term abuse of alcohol induces cycles of damage and repair in the liver, with increased cell turnover. As with the cyclical changes in the breast, this continual increased activity serves to magnify the harm done by the DNA-damaging agents which must also be present, increasing the opportunity for accumulation of further DNA damage and the development of cancer.

As mentioned in Chapter 1, in the case of liver cancer, we also have detailed knowledge of the most frequent carcinogen – hepatitis B infection. The disease is a massive cause of suffering worldwide, but particularly in China and other parts of Asia where up to 10% of the population is chronically infected. There are lower rates in India and the Middle East, with rates less than 1% in Europe and North America. The risk of developing chronic infection is highest in those infected in infancy. Since 1982, a vaccine to HBV has been available. With vaccine programmes in place in various countries for some years, this has allowed scientists to complete the final test of the link between a virus and cancer – if the link were causal, preventing infection should and did prevent the disease. The precise molecular mechanism whereby the virus causes cancer is still being studied, but, as with smoking, the evidence for causation is now compelling.

Moving on to another cancer linked to infection – cervical cancer – we can see a similar story emerging. It was observed in the 1920s that cervical cancer was more common in women who had had high numbers of sexual partners, in particular prostitutes, and it was rare in nuns (except for those who had been previously sexually active), suggesting an infective, sexually transmitted cause. The disease was shown to be linked to infection with the human papillomavirus (HPV) by Harald Zur Hausen in 1976. Dr Zur Hausen found HPV DNA in both genital warts and cervical cancer. He received the Nobel Prize for Medicine for this discovery and his subsequent work in the field, which demonstrated the precise molecular links between the virus and the cancer. The virus produces various proteins which interact with two genes called Rb and p53, both key controllers of the cell cycle, providing an obvious route for generating a cancer.

The development of a vaccine against HPV and hence cervical cancer has proved more technically challenging than the HBV vaccine. However, the linkage between chronic viral infection and cancer allowed the study of the pre-malignant stages of cervical cancer. This led to the discovery that these could be identified in smears of cells taken with a wooden spatula from the cervix and then examined under the microscope. Identification of the pre-cancer stage, called cervical intra-epithelial neoplasia (CIN) or carcinoma-in-situ (CIS), allowed preventative treatment. Most European and North American countries have comprehensive screening based on the cervical smear test. These programmes have been estimated to have saved many thousands of lives. More recently, a vaccine against the varieties of HPV linked to cervical cancer became available in 2006 and is beginning to appear in public health vaccine programmes for girls as a way of preventing infection, with consequent reduction in cancer risk. There is some controversy about the vaccine as some interpret it as a way of protecting against the risks of promiscuity. However, protection against one sexually transmitted disease does not lower risks from others such as HIV. In addition, the vaccine will protect women against the risks of prior promiscuity in their partners, something they have no control over whatsoever. It will, however, take 10 to 20 years for this benefit to be seen, as this is the typical time lag between HPV infection and the development of cancer.

Chapter 3
How is cancer treated?

Cancer treatment is complex and typically will involve input from a number of different groups, ranging from a wide assortment of doctors, including general practitioners (family doctors), surgeons, oncologists, pathologists, radiologists, palliative care specialists, as well as a huge number of other trained personnel – nurses, radiographers, physiotherapists, technicians in laboratories and radiotherapy departments, theatre orderlies, the list goes on and on. The details of organization for these different groups vary enormously from country to country and are a function of both the politics and economics of healthcare.

To try and get around this problem, I will present the organization of cancer treatment as a journey from symptoms to diagnosis, treatment, follow-up, and palliative care for those experiencing incurable recurrence. Different healthcare systems will process these events in a variety of ways, but by and large, the underlying principles are pretty universal. The final part of the chapter gives an overview of the main different classes of treatment, such as surgery, chemotherapy, and radiotherapy.

Initial diagnosis and investigations

Most patients still present with symptoms such as a persistent cough or problems such as blood appearing in the urine. Significant numbers are also picked up by screening programmes, either organized on a systematic basis (for example, for breast and cervical cancer) or more informally (such as PSA testing for prostate cancer). Some cases are picked up as incidental findings in the course of investigation for some other problem. For example, an abdominal scan may detect an asymptomatic tumour in a kidney. I will return to these groups of patients later.

Most patients will present to their doctor with some sort of symptom they have noticed and which they are worried about. Although symptoms, like people, come in an unlimited number of varieties, they can mostly be grouped into those causing disruption of normal function, such as a brain tumour disrupting normal movement, or abnormal symptoms due to damage by the tumour, such as bleeding, pain, or cough. The period between initial symptoms and diagnosis of cancer may be very short or may sometimes run to years. Sometimes the delay in diagnosis is down to misinterpretation of symptoms by health professionals, sometimes deliberate self-neglect or self-deception by patients, and sometimes a mixture of the two.

Unsurprisingly, the perception that an opportunity to make an early diagnosis has been missed can cause severe subsequent problems in the relationship between the patient and their doctor, often at a time when they need them most. Family doctors have a tough time in this respect. For example, headache and backache are common symptoms, and in the vast majority of cases have benign causes that may need symptomatic remedies but do not need extensive investigation. Occasionally, of course, these symptoms may indicate an underlying brain or spinal tumour. Another example is the presence of blood in the bowel motions. All medical students know that this may indicate bowel cancer. All family doctors will know that for patients in the 'at risk' age range for bowel cancer, the presence of conditions like haemorrhoids (an irritating condition of the lower anus that can bleed) are virtually universal. How do they then set about distinguishing the banal from the severe (but rare) without grossly over-investigating their patients? The answer often lies in another basic skill taught in medical school – the art of taking an accurate history. Thus, a sudden and unexpected change such as severe bleeding mixed in with motions is much more likely to be due to a cancer than a small quantity of bright red blood being seen smeared on the toilet paper occurring over a period of years.

Screening for cancer

In an ideal world, we would be able to offer tests that picked up cancer before it reached the more serious stages, allowing early intervention and a much greater prospect of cure. Such a process is called screening and is now available for a number of cancers: breast, uterine, cervix, and bowel. In addition, the PSA blood test is a potential screening test for prostate cancer, but its use remains controversial. It is helpful to describe the characteristics of an ideal screening test and then examine how these tests shape up in practice.

This is illustrated in the following example:

Table 1 - features of an ideal screening test (Source: WHO)

- The target disease should be a common form of cancer, with high associated death rate
- Effective treatment, capable of reducing the risk of death if applied early enough, should be available
- Test procedures should be acceptable, safe, and relatively inexpensive

In addition, we need to consider:

- True positive rates: Sick people correctly diagnosed as sick
- False positive rates: Healthy people wrongly identified as sick
- True negative rates: Healthy people correctly identified as healthy
- False negative rates: Sick people wrongly identified as healthy

---

Table 2. Relation between results of liver scan and correct diagnosis

	Patients with the liver disease	Patients with no liver disease	Totals
Liver scan			
Abnormal (+)	231	32	263
Normal (-)	27	54	81
Totals	258	86	344

Thus the sensitivity (Patients with liver disease and abnormal scans/all patients with a positive scan) = 231/231+31 = 0.88
and the specificity (Patients with normal scans and no disease/all patients with normal scans) = 54/(27+54) = 0.67
A further measure is the positive predictive value (the proportion of patients with abnormal scans who have liver disease) = 231/(231+27) = 0.89
and the negative predictive value of a negative scan (the proportion of patients with normal scans who have no liver disease)
= 54/(32+86) = 0.45

For a test in the clinic, this is pretty good – a positive scan in someone suspected of having liver disease is a pretty good indicator that the person has the disease. How does this fare as a screening test, then?

To illustrate the difference between using a test for diagnosis in someone already known to be ill and screening for disease in people with no symptoms, we can look at the figures for breast cancer. Let us suppose that the rate of missed cases (the specificity) in those who we test is 10% and that the level of early, undetected disease is 1 in 500 people. If we now test 100,000 subjects, an ideal test would yield 200 positive tests in the cancer sufferers and 999,800 negative tests in those without the disease. However, our test, though good, is not perfect and will only detect 180 of the 200 cases, leaving 20 people wrongly reassured. Conversely, the test is also not completely specific. Let us say that 95% of those without the disease will test negative but 5% will wrongly test positive. When we apply this to our screening population, we see that this means that 5% of the 99,800 without the disease will falsely test positive. This works out as 4,990 false positive tests in people without the disease. This means that only a

48

minority (180/4,990 = 4%) of those with a positive test actually have the disease, but 4,990 - 180 = 4,810 people have had a nasty scare. Furthermore, 20 have been falsely reassured and will go on to present with cancer anyway, possibly detected late as they may ignore the symptoms, believing themselves to be cancer-free. However, the overwhelming majority of those with a negative test (99,800 - more than 99%) really were free of the disease, so a negative test is pretty reassuring.

These worked examples are important, as they illustrate the limitations of screening tests which at first sight sound pretty good. In point of fact, the figures above are the *best* figures available – sensitivity and specificity fall in younger women (probably because their breast tissue is denser, making it harder to see abnormal lumps), leading to more incorrectly categorized cases. Furthermore, while the cost of the test itself is small, the cost of chasing up the false positives is much larger and needs to be factored into the costs of the screening programme.

There is a further problem when working out the benefit of screening. In our example above, we will identify cases of cancer earlier than would have happened without screening, potentially improving treatment prospects. However, with breast cancer, the cure rates are good, with three-quarters of diagnosed women being long-term survivors. This leaves the quarter who are destined to do badly, who are the main potential beneficiaries of screening. This is a relatively small number in relation to the numbers of tests carried out, and the downside is over-investigation of healthy women without breast cancer.

Investigating suspected cancer

Whether the patient has been picked up by a screening programme or has presented to their doctor with worrisome

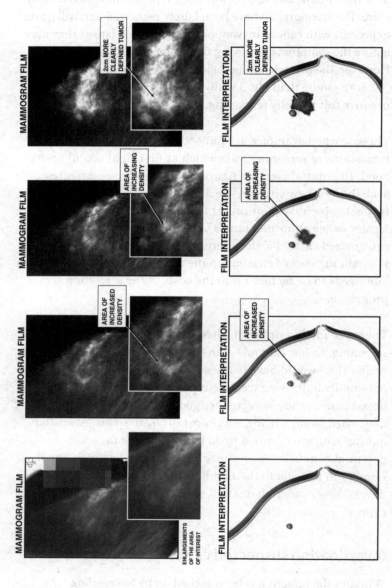

16. Mammogram of breast cancer

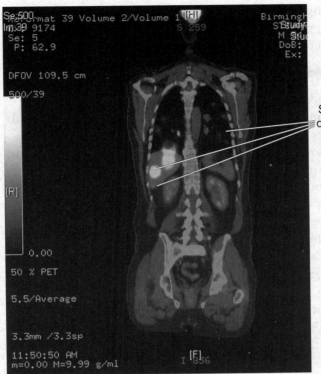

Se:500
Reformat 39 Volume 2/Volume 1 [H]   Birmingh
Im:39 9174   S 259   Study
Se: 5   M Stu
P: 62.9   DoB:
                                              Ex:

DFOV 109.5 cm

500/39

Secondary
deposits of
cancer in
the lungs
and liver

[R]

0.00

50 % PET

5.5/Average

3.3mm /3.3sp

11:50:50 AM
m=0.00 M=9.99 g/ml   [F]
                         I 856

17. Combined CT/PET (positron emission tomography) image of patient with advanced cancer with spread to lungs and liver

symptoms, the next step is to carry out further tests to confirm or exclude the diagnosis. Diagnosis is usually based on a tissue sample (biopsy) of the affected organ, preceded by clinical examination by a doctor, imaging, and blood tests. Ideally, cancer would be investigated using non-invasive imaging tests. In practice, in almost all cases the diagnosis needs to be confirmed by examining a tissue sample in the laboratory. Imaging is key to deciding where and how to obtain tissue. Modern cross-sectional imaging either with X-rays – computed tomography, or CT, scans – or using magnetic resonance imaging (MRI) can give remarkably detailed pictures of internal organs and suspected tumours. However, even the best imaging is unable to show with certainty whether a mass is cancerous and also, even if the diagnosis of cancer is highly likely, exactly what sort of cancer. Occasionally the imaging is sufficient. For example, an elderly, frail, life-long heavy smoker with suspected lung cancer on a chest X-ray and who is unfit for any treatment may be spared the discomfort of a confirming biopsy. One or two other scenarios may also not require a biopsy – patients with extensive cancer deposits in bone (a common site of spread for prostate cancer) on imaging and a grossly elevated serum prostate specific antigen (PSA) can be reliably diagnosed as having widespread prostate cancer with no biopsy. The illustrations show specimen scans of a cancer in the breast (Figure 16) and secondary tumour deposits in the lung and liver (Figure 17). In all of these cases, the abnormalities are evident. However, even for radiologically obvious lesions such as these, a biopsy is generally required to determine the exact cancer type and hence the appropriate treatment.

The role of the pathologist in cancer diagnosis

The pathologist assesses small tissue samples taken, for example, via a needle – biopsies. Occasionally, for example in renal cancer, the initial material may be from a surgically removed organ, such as the diseased kidney. Mostly, this is done by mounting very thin slices of the removed tumour on slides and then carrying out a range of stains which highlight particular features of interest. The stained slides are then examined by the pathologist using a microscope. A commonly used stain is haematoxylin and eosin (usually called H&E) which highlights the various components of the cell such as the nucleus. Increasingly specialized stains are used which help further characterize the tumour. An example would be staining for the oestrogen receptor in breast cancer which helps predict the response of the cancer to both chemotherapy and hormone therapy. There are a rapidly growing number of available tests, mostly based on monoclonal antibodies (which are also increasing rapidly as a form of treatment – see below). In addition, tests can also be done to look for changes in the expression of particular genes or to look for the presence of particular mutations or rearrangements in chromosomes.

The primary question for the pathologist is: 'is it cancer?' If the answer is 'yes', then secondary questions include the specific type – in other words, in which organ did it start and which subtype. In addition, cancers are graded in terms of aggressiveness, typically on a scale of one (low) to three (high). Some cancers, for example prostate cancer, lymphoma (cancer of the lymph glands), and sarcomas (cancers of the connecting and structural tissues such as bone, muscle, or cartilage), have different grading systems, but the same principles apply. All of these systems are based on the size and shape of the cancer cells and how they compare to the normal cells in the organ in which they originated.

More recently, and increasingly, additional subclassification is based on molecular markers present on the cancer. These can be defined as characteristic features based on excessive levels of particular markers either in the tumour itself or circulating in blood (or sometimes present in urine). Probably the best-known example of a molecular marker is HER2 in breast cancer. This was initially described as a marker of poor outcome in breast and ovarian cancer by Dr Denis Slamon from UCLA in the late 1980s. This led to the development of the drug trastuzumab (Herceptin), intended to target cells with excessive amounts of the protein (termed over-expression). Landmark trials, initially in patients with advanced disease and subsequently in newly diagnosed patients, showed that the drug significantly improved outcomes for the 25% of women with tumours with high levels of the HER2 protein. Staining tumour samples for HER2 expression thus gives important information about prognosis (treatment outcomes) and also helps guide the choice of treatment.

The other major role for the pathologist in cancer care is the assessment of specimens resulting from surgical removal of organs containing cancer. In addition to the questions posed above, which will be reassessed with the larger specimen, the pathologist is also addressing issues such as:

• is the tumour confined to the organ that has been removed at surgery?
• are the surgical resection margins (the edges of the specimen) free of tumour?
• is there spread to other associated structures such as lymph glands?

Treatment decision-making

Having carried out a biopsy and appropriate imaging, a decision has to be made about the treatment approach for the patient. An important initial decision is whether or not cure is feasible. If treatment is going to be essentially palliative, this must be factored into decision-making – quality of life becomes paramount. If treatment is potentially curative, then different considerations apply – research has shown that patients will endure considerable side effects in return for a chance of cure. Whether the aim is cure, life prolongation, or palliation of symptoms, a range of approaches are available and may be used either alone or in combination. Decisions need to be reviewed on a regular basis and treatment adapted in accordance with side effects and tumour response – that is, whether or not things are improving.

Increasingly, in major healthcare systems, these decisions are not made by individual doctors but by a multi-disciplinary team, usually abbreviated to MDT (in the UK, this is now mandatory if the hospital is to receive reimbursement for cancer therapy). Typically, these teams will comprise surgeons, radiation and medical oncologists, radiologists, pathologists, and specialist nurses. The MDT will review the baseline information (termed staging information) prior to the consultation with the patient to review the various test results. Generally, these decisions will be based on national or international guidelines on best practice. The results and treatment options will then be discussed with the patient in the clinic, and the clinical plan finalized.

The various treatment modalities will be dealt with in turn, but before doing so, it may be helpful to give a broad breakdown of the relative importance of the treatment modalities. Figure 18 gives an estimate of how 100 'typical' patients would be treated in a modern Western healthcare system. Clearly, the numbers are for illustration only and will vary by country, and even within countries with local practice. For example, bladder cancer can be managed either by surgery to remove the bladder (cystectomy) or by radiotherapy to destroy the tumour, with surgery reserved for salvage of radiotherapy failures. In the USA, very few patients are managed electively with radiotherapy, which is reserved mostly for palliation (symptom control) in the elderly and frail. In contrast, in the UK, around two-thirds of patients are managed with primary radiotherapy, with surgery focused on the younger, fitter patients. These differences in practice stem largely from the differences in the

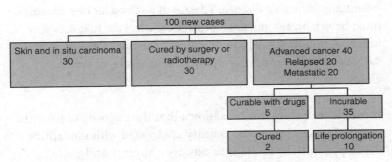

18. Distribution of cancer care between treatment modalities

UK and US health economies (see Chapter 5) rather than any evidence-driven differences.

The essential principle underlying the distribution is that around 30% of cases are only very locally invasive – for example, basal skin cancers (commonly called rodent ulcers) – and require a very limited local therapy, usually surgery but occasionally radiotherapy. Of the rest, around 40% of patients end up with widespread cancer and 30% have locally advanced cancer, which can be eradicated by local/regional treatments such as surgery or radiotherapy. As already indicated, the precise split varies in part by geography but also varies with anatomical site. For example, cancer of the colon is best treated with surgery rather than radiotherapy, as a normal large bowel is relatively intolerant of radiotherapy, and also targeting a mobile structure is clearly problematical. On the other hand, cancer of the uterine cervix (neck of the womb) is now predominantly treated by radiotherapy combined with simultaneous chemotherapy, with surgery reserved for salvage cases plus a limited role in assessing the disease for local spread.

Of the patients who end up with advanced cancer, around half present with this in the first place, the other half start out with apparently localized disease but then subsequently relapse with more widespread problems. Of patients who develop advanced (usually called metastatic) cancer, the majority will have essentially incurable disease. These will be diseases like advanced lung, bowel, breast, prostate, or liver cancer – the major cancer killers. A minority will have potentially chemocurable diseases such as testicular cancer, lymphoma, leukaemia, or certain childhood cancers.

It can be seen from this breakdown that the majority of patients cured of cancer in the 21st century are treated with modalities developed initially in the 19th century – surgery and radiotherapy. The major drug treatment advances, which drive so many of the news headlines, started in the mid-20th century and mostly extend lives in advanced disease rather than actually curing patients. This fact is well known to public health doctors but less well appreciated by the general public. It follows from this that in poorer economies, the maximum impact on cancer will be obtained by putting in place good basic surgery and radiotherapy. The best illustration of this is the survival rates worldwide for rectal cancer, for which the best results are obtained in Cuba, renowned for its well-organized medical care but with very limited access to the more expensive new drugs. Where resources are limited, cancer chemotherapy is best focused on the rare chemocurable cancers such as childhood leukaemia and testicular cancer. As these cancers mostly occur in younger people, the impact from drug spend in this area on life years saved is disproportionately high compared to spending on end-of-life cancer drugs in older patients. Drug therapy for advanced disease occurring in later life tends to have a much smaller impact on cure rates. Even if cures were common, the patients themselves are older and thus have more limited life expectancy anyway. This topic will be dealt with in more detail in Chapter 5.

Surgery

Surgery clearly dates back millennia, but the era of cancer surgery really dates back to the development of effective anaesthesia in the mid-19th century, which moved surgery from the ghastly, last-ditch 'gore-fest' of emergency amputations to controlled dissections. As already discussed, surgery to remove the tumour is one of the mainstays of cancer therapy (together with radiotherapy), and despite advances in drug treatment seems set to remain so for the foreseeable future. Increasingly, surgeons are developing minimally invasive (often called keyhole) techniques to operate without performing large incisions. These have the advantage of rapid postoperative recovery, but do increase operation times and are technically challenging. These techniques do allow older, frailer patients to be operated on due to the faster recovery times. They are also more generally attractive to all patient groups as they are less painful in the recovery period and rehabilitation to full normal function is quicker. Against this, operating via long metal tubes whilst peering down a modified telescope has been likened to tying your shoelaces with chopsticks, making exponents of open surgery claim that the key cancer outcomes – completeness of tumour

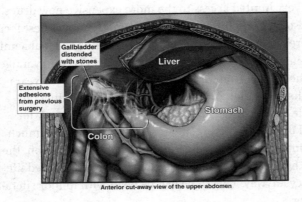

Anterior cut-away view of the upper abdomen

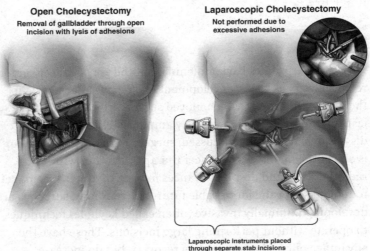

Open Cholecystectomy
Removal of gallbladder through open incision with lysis of adhesions

Laparoscopic Cholecystectomy
Not performed due to excessive adhesions

Laparoscopic instruments placed through separate stab incisions

19. Comparison of open and laparoscopic gall bladder removal

removal, for example – may be compromised. Assessment of this aspect of care is made by the pathologist – a key member of the cancer team.

A recent development in minimal access surgery is the robot-assisted procedure. In a robotic operation, the instruments are inserted manually and then fixed into the robot arms. Viewing ports are inserted and the surgeon operates at a console separate from the patient – essentially using computer games technology to manipulate the instruments remotely. There are potential downsides to this exciting technology – for example, the set-up time for the robot instruments is longer than directly manipulated 'keyhole' instruments. Also, the machines themselves cost around £1,000,000 to buy and approximately £150,000 per year to run. This is a considerable additional outlay over and above all the general infrastructure of operating theatres, wards, anaesthetic departments, and so on. Whether ultimately this will turn out to be both clinically and cost effective clearly remains to be seen. Certainly in the USA, there is now very strong consumer/patient

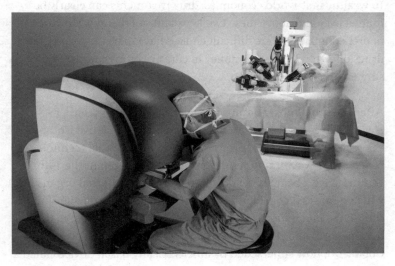

20. **Robot-assisted surgery**

demand for robotic surgery that may ultimately override the colder clinical considerations.

Radiotherapy

Radiotherapy is another 19th-century technology still going strong in the 21st century. Roentgen made the key observations underpinning modern radiotherapy in 1895 when he observed that invisible rays (which he called 'X-rays') were produced when electrons were fired at a target in a vacuum – revealed by their ability to blacken photographic film. It was rapidly realized that X-rays were transmitting energy and that this energy could be potentially focused for treatment as well as imaging. Within a matter of months, the first patients with skin tumours were treated – a breathtaking rate of innovation. The technologies of both imaging and therapy have gradually been refined and improved over the last century or so, and now form key components of modern cancer therapy. Indeed, as already noted, the most effective parts of modern cancer therapy remain surgery and radiotherapy, with the additional gain from drug treatment in terms of cure rates being relatively marginal. In wealthy first-world economies, drug treatments can clearly be funded over and above these two key planks of therapy. However, in poorer countries, where difficult choices have to be made, very few drugs offer good value for money in curative terms compared to surgery and radiotherapy.

After the initial observations of the effects of X-rays, either electrically generated or produced by using radioactive isotopes, the technology has been progressively refined. Initial technology based on the vacuum tubes described by Roentgen in the 19th century gave a beam which could penetrate to internal organs but which deposited considerably more of the dose nearer the skin. In the 1950s, much more powerful, so-called mega-voltage machines became available. These were based on the artificial isotope Cobalt-60, now superseded by an electrically based device called a linear accelerator, usually abbreviated to linac. These latter machines used the magnetron valve developed in the Second World War for radar. The pulsed energy can be used to 'shove' electrons into the target at much higher energies with much better properties for treating deep-seated tumours – a sort of electronic ploughshare from a high-tech sword.

Modern radiotherapy can be very precisely targeted by integrating treatment delivery with detailed imaging. Side effects arise in two ways. In structures such as skin, gut lining, and the mouth, the effects can be likened to sunburn, with severity depending on the dose received. Effects experienced depend on the site treated and may include diarrhoea with lower bowel treatment, or sore mouth, hair loss, and reddening in treated skin, and so on. A second group of side effects is experienced in solid structures such as lung and kidney. In these organs, there is little immediate effect, but if critical dose constraints are exceeded, the irradiated tissue will progressively fail. Dose to critical organs adjacent to the target tumour is thus a key restriction on the delivery of radiotherapy – a certain amount of toxicity will be worth accepting in order to treat the cancer, but clearly there comes a point when the damage may outweigh the benefit. Improved radiotherapy such as intensity-modulated radiotherapy (IMRT), involving very sophisticated dose distributions which appear to 'bend' dose around critical structures, is increasingly becoming available but increases costs and complexity of delivery. A linked development is on-board imaging in treatment machines which can be used to give image-guided radiotherapy (IGRT) where the treatment tracks movements in the tumour from day to day. The combination of IMRT and IGRT has the potential to both increase tumour control (by ensuring treatment is on target) and decrease side effects by better sparing of uninvolved tissues.

Hormone therapy

Although chemotherapy now dominates cancer drug therapy, it was a hormone-based drug therapy that was the first successful medicinal cancer treatment. Hormone therapy for cancer dates back to the 1940s following observations made by Charles Huggins, an American urologist, on patients with advanced prostate cancer.

The pioneers of hormone therapy reasoned that if the 'parent' tissue needed normal hormone levels, then the abnormal tumour derived from the tissue may retain this dependence. Trials of castration in advanced prostate cancer produced dramatic results, with rapid and substantial improvements in symptoms such as pain from cancer deposits in bone. Following this, administration of female hormones, which of course suppress male characteristics, was attempted, again with dramatic results. Sadly, these endocrine effects, while substantial, would last for only 1 or 2 years, the disease then recurring. Similar effects were observed in pre-menopausal women with breast cancer following removal of the ovaries. The subsequent decades have seen the development of a whole range of hormone-based medications for both prostate cancer and breast cancer in particular. One of these drugs, the oestrogen blocker tamoxifen, is probably responsible for saving more lives than any other anticancer drug. More than half a century on, new drugs targeting the hormone pathways are still appearing in the clinic.

Chemotherapy

If members of the public are asked to name the class of drugs most associated with cancer treatment, they will say chemotherapy. The term covers a wide range of different agents with diverse origins from antibiotics to plant extracts to synthetic chemicals based on DNA. All interfere with the mechanics of cell division and, as many tissues have dividing cells, this leads to the typical side effects such as nausea and vomiting (partly from damage to the gut lining, partly from a direct effect on the brain), hair loss (damage to hair follicles), and risk of infection (damage to the production of white blood cells needed to defend against infection). We are all familiar with the images of billiard-ball bald patients 'fighting' cancer (to use the tabloid press term). Whilst this does occur with chemotherapy, the reality is more varied, with much chemotherapy given in the outpatient setting producing little nausea or hair loss. Hair loss is hard to prevent, but it is not a uniform property of all chemotherapy drugs. Nausea and vomiting are now pretty largely preventable, allowing the administration of drugs hitherto considered too toxic, even to quite elderly patients. This is important because much chemotherapy is given for palliation of symptoms, hence quality of life is of paramount importance. There is arguably little point to life prolongation if the quality of that life is poor.

The first chemotherapy drugs were based on chemicals derived from mustard gas, used extensively to ghastly effect in the First World War. It was noted that soldiers exposed to these agents who survived would experience drops in their white blood cells (the cells in the blood that are responsible for defence against infection). There is, of course, a cancer of the white blood cells – usually termed leukaemia. Trials were carried out of mustard gas derivatives such as mustine in both leukaemia and a second related group of cancers called lymphoma. Patients in these trials experienced for the first time remissions of what had previously been untreatable conditions. With drugs used singly, unfortunately these remissions turned out to be temporary. However, further drugs followed, and trials established that using these drugs in combinations could lead to cures for patients with leukaemia and lymphoma.

A wave of new chemotherapy drugs followed, and in the 1970s and 1980s it was widely assumed that these would in turn lead to curative therapies for most cases of advanced cancer. These drugs came from a variety of sources. Plant extracts (vincristine, docetaxel, paclitaxel), complexed heavy metals (cisplatinum, carboplatin), and antibiotics (doxorubicin, mitomycin) proved to be fruitful areas of discovery leading to large-scale laboratory screening programmes looking for promising chemicals in a whole range of plant and bacterial extracts. Another area of discovery was compounds derived from the components of DNA or other building blocks of the cell division process, the best example being 5-fluoro-uracil, which is a derivative of uracil, one of the components of RNA (see Chapter 2). The extra fluorine atom in the molecule allows 5FU to interact with DNA and RNA but not to be processed normally – a molecular 'spanner' in the works.

In the 1970s and 1980s, further notable successes followed, in particular advanced testicular cancer was transformed from a lethal to a highly curable condition. The magnitude of this success is best illustrated by seven-times Tour de France champion Lance Armstrong who was diagnosed with very extensive disease, including brain involvement. After successful extensive chemotherapy, he went on to win his first Tour, followed by a record-breaking six further triumphs. Similar successes have been seen in the leukaemias and a range of childhood cancers. Sadly, however, the major cancer killers have proved to be more resistant to chemotherapy, with cures elusive, although most tumour types will respond to chemotherapy to a degree. It was suggested that the problem may have been that insufficiently large doses of chemotherapy were being given. However, a round of trials in the 1990s showed that even extreme doses of combination chemotherapy together with a bone marrow transplant were unable to cure major killers such as advanced breast cancer.

This realization has led to a change of emphasis. The observation that advanced disease, while incurable, would respond to chemotherapy for a while led to the testing of chemotherapy in the setting of early disease, as had previously been done with hormone therapy. It was known that many patients with no obvious disease nonetheless later developed recurrence. This suggested that there must be very small amounts of cancer lurking undetected. The hypothesis was that giving chemotherapy early may work better than waiting for detectable relapse. Initial trials were disappointing but with hindsight were simply too small to detect the benefits. When trial results were pooled in breast cancer, it was realized that there was a benefit to early chemotherapy, with women receiving it relapsing later and surviving longer compared to those for whom chemotherapy was saved as a 'salvage' treatment. This is called adjuvant therapy and works on the principle that so-called 'micro-metastatic' disease may be eradicable, whereas once the disease is visible on a scan it is incurable. Essentially, modern scanners, whilst very sensitive, are unable to detect tumours smaller than a few millimetres across. Hence we cannot distinguish between people who have been cured by initial surgery or radiotherapy and those who have apparently normal scans but in reality harbour small residual tumour deposits destined to cause relapse in the future. Subsequent studies have refined the drug combinations used and also the groups of women deriving most benefit. The problem with adjuvant therapy is that many women will do well just with surgery and radiotherapy, and thus derive no benefit from the chemotherapy, only toxicity and potential harm. This risk is greatest for those with lowest risk of disease recurrence, either due to less aggressive disease or high risk of death from other causes (for example, the very elderly).

More recently, greater emphasis has been placed on the role of chemotherapy in palliation of symptoms. This may seem like an oxymoron – giving toxic drugs to reduce suffering. However, improved symptom control, in particular with drugs that prevent the severe nausea previously associated with chemotherapy, has transformed the value of these agents for palliation. The survival gains seen are often relatively modest – typically a matter of months – leading to researchers developing methods for measuring quality of life. This allows comparison of toxic drugs producing benefit, for example by reducing pain, with alternatives often described under the blanket term of 'best supportive care' – painkillers, radiotherapy, and so on.

These two trends – adjuvant and palliative use – have greatly increased the cancer drug bill in the developed world (see Chapter 5) as, although the gains are relatively small, the numbers who can benefit are enormous, and this has resulted in widespread use of chemotherapy in relatively elderly cancer patients.

Monoclonal antibodies

Antibodies are a key component of the body's immune defences. Each antibody comprises a constant region and a variable region. The variable region is responsible for the binding of the antibody to its target – this is illustrated in Figure 21. The normal function of antibodies is to bind to invading infectious organisms – viruses, bacteria, and so on. When exposed to a new infection, the body's white blood cells identify it and select the cells (called lymphocytes) with the antibody-variable region best able to stick to and disable the invader. Production of the relevant cells is massively increased, followed by increased production of antibodies able to bind to the invader. Once bound, other immune cells identify the antibody-coated invaders and ingest them, using the antibody-constant region as a 'hook' for pulling them out of the circulation. The development of an immune system is one of the key evolutionary steps necessary for the existence of complex multicellular organisms. Those born with inherited defects in their immune systems struggle to survive childhood, underlining the importance of this function.

In the 1970s, technology was developed to exploit the ability of the immune system by manufacturing antibodies against 'artificial' targets such as cancer cells. These engineered targeted antibodies are called monoclonal antibodies – antibodies made by a single clone of cells – and can be made to stick to pretty much any chosen target. By picking targets on cancer cells, these natural molecules can be used both as an aid to imaging, by linkage to radioactive chemicals, or simply as treatments in their own right.

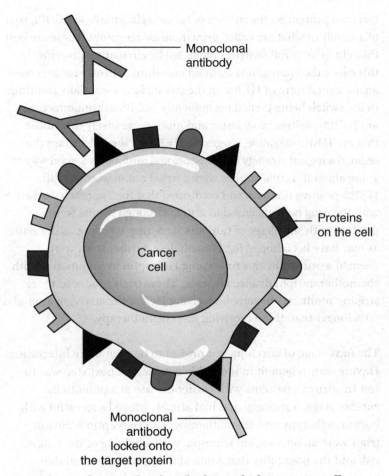

Monoclonal
antibody

Proteins
on the cell

Cancer
cell

Monoclonal
antibody
locked onto
the target protein

21. Diagram of a monoclonal antibody attached to a cancer cell

When they first appeared, it was thought that monoclonal antibodies would be the 'magic bullet' that would eradicate advanced cancer by being custom-made to order for each tumour. The reality sadly proved to be less dramatic, but 30 years on, monoclonal antibodies are now hitting the clinics in increasing numbers.

The best-known monoclonal antibody is probably trastuzumab, more often referred to by its trade name of Herceptin. The drug targets a protein on the surface of cancer cells known as HER2, part of a family of what are called growth factor receptors. These are best thought of as on/off switches regulated by circulating proteins (in this case called heregulin). Around one-third of breast cancers have an abnormal form of HER2 on the cell surface, essentially resulting in the switch being turned permanently 'on'. Breast tumours that are HER2-positive grow faster and more aggressively than those that are HER2-negative. Targeting HER2 on the cell surface thus seemed a logical strategy and monoclonal antibodies a good way of going about it. Initial studies were carried out in women with HER2-positive tumours and confirmed that the approach worked, with the drug being licensed in 2002. Although results were positive, with shrinkage of tumours seen, they were not as dramatic as may have been hoped for. Nonetheless, further trials were deemed worthwhile, this time using Herceptin in conjunction with chemotherapy for advanced disease. These trials produced more striking results, with women receiving Herceptin surviving around 50% longer than those receiving just chemotherapy.

The next stage of development proved to be even more interesting. Having shown benefit in incurable disease, the next step was to test the drug in patients with earlier disease at a potentially curable stage, a strategy that had already proved successful with hormone therapy and chemotherapy. The Herceptin adjuvant trials were an oncological triumph, with a halving of the relapse risk and the possibility that some of the previously incurable women were actually cured. There was a catch, however. Most women with early HER2-positive breast cancer actually already had a good outlook just with surgery, radiotherapy, and chemotherapy. If a woman is already cured by these treatments, she clearly cannot benefit from any further treatment (and may indeed be harmed, as Herceptin carries a risk of heart disease).

Conversely, some women will still die despite all current therapies, and therefore they too will benefit relatively little. In between are the real winners, converted from those destined to relapse to those potentially cured. This means that in the adjuvant (preventative) setting, the number needed who must be treated to benefit one of the real winners is high, maybe as many as 20. As the cost of Herceptin is substantial (around £30,000 per year), the effective cost per woman saved can be estimated as around 20 x 30,000 = £600,000. Unsurprisingly, therefore, when the drug was licensed for adjuvant use, a further storm of controversy followed – how much is it reasonable to spend to save one life?

Targeted molecular therapies

The DNA revolution and the sequencing of the entire human genome always promised that the benefits would result in better medicines. As more and more genes were cloned, it became possible to map the genes that were abnormal in cancer cells compared to normal cells. Once a key gene is identified, it then became possible to design drugs to target the abnormal gene or, more precisely, its associated protein product. One way to target therapies is with antibodies, as described above. The other way, now generating large numbers of new drugs, is to produce chemicals that interfere with the function, either of the abnormal protein itself or of one of the other elements of the same pathway in the cell. The first and probably best example of the first strategy is the leukaemia drug imatinib (Glivec). A form of leukaemia called chronic lymphocytic leukaemia (CLL) has long been known to be characterized by the presence of a so-called 'Philadelphia chromosome'. This abnormal chromosome is a fusion of two different chromosomes and results in the production of an abnormal protein derived from two different genes – called the bcr-abl fusion protein. Detailed molecular biology studies established that bcr-abl was both necessary and sufficient (the key conditions for a candidate new drug development) to drive the CLL cells, making it an ideal target. The drug imatinib was the first drug to successfully hit the target and it transformed the prognosis for CLL, with prolonged remissions occurring in patients resistant to the chemotherapy drugs previously used. Sadly, however, the remissions, while lengthy, were not permanent – the cancer cells eventually became resistant. This has been a feature of the targeted small molecular therapies – they are often exquisitely effective, with low side effects compared to chemotherapy, but generally do not lead to cures. However, as already noted in the chemotherapy section with leukaemia, initial use of these drugs singly also only produced remissions but not cures, so hopefully combination use will prove similarly beneficial. Time will tell.

The second approach to targeted therapy is to aim for the pathway that is linked to the 'core' abnormality. The best example of this is the recent transformation of kidney cancer therapy. Until recently, advanced kidney cancer was all but untreatable, with only two drugs licensed, interferon and interleukin-2, both of very limited effectiveness. Most kidney cancers occur 'spontaneously', that is to say, no other family members develop the same cancer. It had been observed many years ago that rare families developed the same tumours, often at a very young age – see the section in Chapter 2 on inherited cancer. One such inherited syndrome was described by von Hippel and Lindau and now bears their names. Patients with von Hippel Lindau (VHL) syndrome develop multiple early kidney cancers as part of the disease. Microscopically, the VHL cancers resembled the much more common, non-inherited cancers, so it was suspected that abnormalities in the VHL gene may be present in the spontaneous cancers, and this did indeed turn out to be the case. However, the problem in patients with VHL syndrome is that the normal function in the VHL protein is *missing*; hence targeting the VHL protein itself would only make the problem worse. Study of the VHL pathway revealed that as a result of VHL underactivity, proteins normally suppressed by the VHL protein became overactive. These include proteins driving the cells to divide and a further family of molecules driving the production of new blood vessels. Drugs were developed which targeted members of this pathway, either up- or downstream of the misfiring VHL protein, including three small molecular therapies, sunitinib, sorafenib, and temsirolimus, and a monoclonal antibody called bevacizumab.

Trials of these drugs have resulted in the treatment of advanced kidney cancer being revolutionized, with all four drugs licensed since 2006 and a further raft of additional drugs also heading into the clinic. As with CLL, however, although for the first time large advanced tumours could be made to shrink, the drugs do not result in cures in most cases, and treatment resistance develops with time. Trials are now focusing on adjuvant therapy, sequencing, and combinations in the hope that further survival gains can be made.

As with the Herceptin story above, the drugs have caused huge controversy due to their cost – patients need to be treated continuously rather than with a limited course of treatment, as was previously the norm with treatments such as chemotherapy. The drugs are expensive – around £25,000–£30,000 per year of treatment – with consequent variations in access (see Chapter 5). Unlike with Herceptin and breast cancer, however, purchasing authorities in a range of countries, including Canada, Australia, Scotland, and England, have been more resistant to funding treatments for a group of predominantly elderly male patients than they were for the very vocal women's breast cancer lobby.

Drugs used for symptom control

Although not directly treating the cancer, a range of supportive care drugs have contributed to big improvements in cancer treatments over the last 10 to 15 years. The improved anti-sickness drugs have already been mentioned. Also related to chemotherapy safety and delivery are the growth factors, in particular granulocyte colony stimulating factor (G-CSF) which boosts white blood cell counts, reducing infection risks. A second related product called GM-CSF (granulocyte-macrophage colony stimulating factor), initially developed for the same purpose, has turned out to have a valuable role in releasing blood cell precursors called stem cells into the circulation. This somewhat esoteric observation has allowed the harvesting of stem cells prior to high-dose chemotherapy intended to destroy the normal bone marrow. Previously patients needed a bone marrow transplant to 'rescue' them from such treatment, but it turns out that harvested stem cells do the same job but more quickly and with a much easier pre-treatment harvesting procedure, extending the range of patients suitable for these high-dose therapies.

Another area of recent research has been bone-protecting agents. Many cancers spread into bone with devastating consequences, including pain, fracture, and paralysis due to spinal column damage. Research demonstrated that the body 'over-reacting' to the cancer led, paradoxically, to increased damage. Drugs initially developed for osteoporosis (bone thinning) turned out to reduce this collateral, self-inflicted damage. The initial drugs available, such as clodronate, were relatively low in potency but later drugs, such as zoledronate and ibandronate, are many times more effective and can substantially reduce bone damage in patients with advanced cancer. Even more intriguingly, in adjuvant trials in high-risk breast cancer, zoledronate also appeared to reduce soft tissue disease, suggesting these agents may in addition have direct anticancer properties.

Conclusions

The improvements in cancer treatment seen in the last 100 years have been dramatic and have transformed the outcomes for millions of people across the world. Cancer treatment in the early 21st century is safer, more effective, and less toxic than it was 50 or 100 years ago. Surgery and radiotherapy continue to be refined and improved, with better targeting and minimal access technologies increasingly available. The ancillary imaging and pathology services will also continue to improve and allow better selection of treatment options in the future. The range of drugs and the effectiveness of those drugs are increasing rapidly, and this will generate further improvements in the coming years. The main problem with all this, as we shall see in Chapter 5, is the escalating cost, but grappling with this issue is better than not having the options available.

Chapter 4
Cancer research

Introduction

As we have already seen, the mainstays of cancer therapy remain surgery and radiotherapy, both of which date from the 19th century but which have undergone a process of continual technical improvement, which is still ongoing. Drug treatments for cancer are comparatively much more recent. The first successful cancer drug therapy was the use of synthetic female hormones to treat prostate cancer in the 1940s. Successful curative chemotherapy really dates from the 1970s with the development of treatments for leukaemias and lymphomas (cancers of the bone marrow and lymphatic system), although interestingly, the chemicals on which these treatments are based were previously developed for more nefarious purposes (as we have seen, mustine, one of the first successful drugs in this area, is based on the active ingredient of mustard gas). The development of new treatments and the improvement of existing ones clearly requires a process of research. This chapter will describe some of the ways in which research happens, in particular the differences between the rules for drugs and those for devices (such as radiotherapy machines) or techniques (surgery). These contrasts will be explored in some detail, as there are important differences, with significant anomalies resulting. The chapter will focus mostly on where new treatments come from, but similar trial structures apply to testing existing treatments against each other or for research into techniques of symptom control.

The development process for new surgical and radiotherapy techniques differs significantly from that applying to drugs. Typically, a surgical improvement will be a small technical change (for example, a better way to control bleeding) that does not fundamentally conceptually alter the underlying technique. Such improvements are often licensed essentially on a 'fitness for purpose' basis (that is, does it really help control bleeding?). Similar arguments apply to technical radiotherapy improvements (for example, better ways of targeting radiation to spare normal tissues). In general, it has been taken as self-evident that improvements of these sorts must be better and their implementation will follow. In fact, the improvements may be illusory and commercial pressure rather than any sound evidence base may drive their implementation. I will illustrate how and why this may arise using robotic surgical techniques and intensity-modulated radiotherapy as examples.

Drug treatments, on the other hand, have to meet fundamentally different criteria. Generally, an improvement in survival rates compared to the previous standard of care is required by regulatory authorities such as the Food and Drug Administration (FDA) in the USA. This means a new drug treatment requires testing in a series of clinical trials involving large numbers of patients. Broadly, these can be divided into three categories termed phases 1 to 3.

Phase 1 trials establish the safety and side-effect profile of a drug. Typically, these will involve small numbers of patients, for cancer drugs usually those who have run out of standard options and who will have had multiple previous treatments. Drugs with less dramatic effects, for example blood pressure drugs, will often be tested first on healthy volunteers. Phase 2 trials are larger and will often involve patients earlier in the 'cancer journey' than phase 1 studies, and they aim to confirm that a drug has useful activity against the target cancer. For a drug that looks promising, the final phase 3 trial will compare it with whatever is considered the standard of care. A phase 3 trial will involve many hundreds or even thousands of patients. There are a range of problems inherent in this design, ranging from consent and cost to legislative burdens. Phase 3 licensing trials are now almost always international affairs and have to comply with legislative frameworks from multiple countries, in particular the USA. The costs of such trials are enormous and explain the very high costs of new drugs – around $1 billion from synthesis to registration of a new cancer drug. The licensing process – which gives a company the lucrative right to market a drug or product – is tightly regulated by national or transnational bodies such as the FDA. This theme of regulation will be developed further in the next chapter – arguably, the high level of trial regulation protects the individual participant in a trial from possible harm at the expense of society at large by slowing the pace of improvement and driving up the costs of new drugs to the point when access is increasingly restricted, even in the most wealthy of economies.

Developing new cancer drugs

Basic science

Clearly, a massive body of biological research underpins cancer research. There have been huge advances made in the last 50 years, particularly the unravelling of the structure of DNA and the so-called 'central dogma' of biology – the relationship between DNA, RNA, and protein discussed in detail in Chapter 2. Previous generations of cancer drugs were developed largely by observing the effects of chemicals on cells, looking for drugs that were particularly effective at killing cancer cells. This research produced the chemotherapy drugs that appeared in large numbers in the 1970s and 1980s. Although new chemotherapy agents are still being produced, there is a sense of diminishing returns from more recent drugs compared to the huge advances of previous decades.

More recent research has focused on the evolving knowledge of the molecular signatures of cancer discussed in the previous chapter in relation to targeted small molecules and monoclonal antibodies. The human genome was sequenced in the late 20th century. The initial sequencing technology was cumbersome and slow, and the first complete sequence took many years to complete. Having completed this task, and with the overall structure of the human genome now known, it has become possible to sequence the genomes of specific cancers and to compare the cancer DNA to the patient's normal DNA extracted from their blood cells. This now takes teams in specialized laboratories a few weeks and costs are falling rapidly. The technology, time required, and costs are likely to improve dramatically over the next few years such that it will soon be possible to individually determine the DNA sequence of each patient's cancer as part of the diagnostic work-up. For the time being, this work is experimental, and remarkable results are emerging from this new field of study.

The human cell contains around 21,000 genes arranged in 23 chromosomes. Research comparing the DNA sequence of the entire 21,000 genes with the normal DNA of the patients has now been done for a number of cancers, and the results illustrate how small the line is between normal and cancerous cells. On average, experiments of this sort reveal abnormalities in around 40 to 60 genes. Put another way, if we picture the human genome as a library of 23 books (the chromosomes) each of around 1,000 pages (genes), there will be a total of 40 to 60 typographic errors in the entire cancer cell version of the 'library'. Furthermore, many of these genetic 'typos' will not actually alter the 'sense' of the gene – the protein produced will retain normal function. The number of key drivers of the cancer process boils down to around 12 pathways. The genes mutated or misfiring in cancers studied in this way all belong to one of these pathways and appear to be present in all cancers studied. This work points the way to the next stage of cancer drug development. The recent round of small molecules and monoclonals have largely (but not entirely) focused on single molecules such as HER2 being targeted by Herceptin. This recent whole genome work highlights the need to target pathways of multiple genes rather than single members. Drug screens in the future are likely to focus on this aspect of cancer biology, in tandem with whole genome screens to pinpoint the key mutated genes in particular cancers. It also opens the possibility that the drugs of tomorrow will be known to work in the presence of particular genetic signatures. Therefore, linking whole genome sequencing to diagnosis points the way to one of the 'holy grails' of cancer medicine – the personalized selection of drug therapies.

Pre-clinical phase

The first step in the development of new drugs is the identification of suitable compounds for study in human beings. Increasingly, this results from the sort of research work on cancer pathways described above. This search at present can take many forms, from screening of random compounds to the targeted synthesis of drugs to hit pre-specified abnormalities in the cancer cell. The drugs currently used in the clinic come from a range of sources, and some of these have been described in the previous chapter. The initial testing of a candidate drug will involve experiments with cancer cells in the laboratory. These cancer cells come from a variety of sources, ranging from human cancers to artificial tumours generated in laboratory animals. Some of the human cell lines were grown by taking fragments of a surgically removed cancer and placing it in cell culture medium in the laboratory. The process is conceptually attractive – you can test your drug on the 'real' cancer.

There are many such cell lines, possibly the most famous is the HeLa cell line. This was grown from a fragment of cervical cancer taken from a woman called Henrietta Lacks (also sometimes referred to as Helen Lane or Helen Larson in an attempt early on to preserve her privacy), and the cells are very widely used in laboratories around the world. Parenthetically, neither she nor her family gave their consent or permission for this process, resulting in a famous court case in California in 1990 in which it was decided that, in the USA, such a process was lawful. In the UK and other countries, the position is different and informed patient consent for tissue collection is now enforced by legislation. It has been calculated that so many HeLa cells have been cultured that they outnumber many times over the 'normal' cells produced by Ms Lacks in her lifetime, giving her a curious form of immortality. The problem with cell lines, however, is that most attempts to grow tumour cells from patients are unsuccessful. Hence the cell lines we have may be as unrepresentative of the typical cancer as HeLa cells are of the person that was Henrietta Lacks. Nonetheless, despite this limitation, human cancer cell lines remain a key component of cancer research and drug testing.

The second form of cell lines used are derived from animal tumours, mostly arising in mice. Many of these tumours are artificially engineered. A good example of this is an engineered cell line used in prostate cancer research. Mice do not get prostate cancer in the way that humans do. However, it is possible to identify genes that are expressed in mouse prostate and to use the promoter regions (see Chapter 2) of those genes to drive the production of proteins that cause cancer. In the case of mice, a gene with the curious name of 'large-T' from a cancer-causing virus called SV40 is used. Parenthetically, while many genes have names that are strings of unmemorable letters and numbers (there are 21,000 human genes alone after all – a lot to name), a subset have names varying from the odd (large-T) to the odder (hedgehog, notchless) to downright amusing – a pair of genes involved in cell signalling are called 'mad' and 'Max'!

In order to have mice develop prostate tumours, the hybrid gene containing the prostate specific gene promoter and the SV40-T gene must be inserted into a fertilized mouse egg. If the insertion is successful, a transgenic mouse results and the growing mice will now express the foreign gene in their prostate glands. As would be predicted, these mice go on to develop multiple prostate tumours. A number of these cancer-prone mice were bred, and the strain is called the TRansgenic Adenocarcinoma of the Mouse Prostate (TRAMP) model. These mice have proved useful in a number of ways. As the mice reliably develop tumours, they can be used to test cancer-preventing strategies such as dietary interventions. Secondly, the tumours can be used to test drug treatments for effectiveness. Thirdly, tumour cells arising in TRAMP mice have been successfully cultured in the lab and these cell lines can be used for experiments, either alone or re-implanted into adult animals from the same mouse strain – quicker and more reproducible than waiting for the tumours to develop in the TRAMP mice themselves. It is again obvious from the above discussions that such models are only representations of aspects of the human disease, not perfect replications of it. Hence, while useful, drugs must ultimately be tested in humans.

Before a drug can be administered to human subjects, a further phase of pre-clinical testing is required – toxicity testing. While animal models and cell culture provide valuable indications of whether a drug may be active in man, they do not tell us whether it is safe. We also need to know whether it is likely that we can achieve drug levels in patients that will be high enough to realistically have an impact on the cancer. The standard way of exploring this is to give escalating drug doses to groups of animals until we start to see animals dying from drug side effects. There are a number of rather grisly standard measures, such as the dose of drug that will kill a proportion of the test subjects – termed the lethal dose (LD) test. Measures such as LD50 (the dose that kills 50% of the animals) and LD10 (10% death rate) are widely used and attract much controversy from anti-vivisection groups. I don't propose to examine the ethics of animal testing *per se* – it seems to me to be something you believe is right or believe is wrong. If you fall in the latter category, then no amount of argument will generally alter opinions. I do believe it is worth critically examining the scientific basis of animal testing to try and minimize unnecessary suffering. There are many very obvious problems with LD50 testing – for example, the LD50 will vary widely for different species for a given compound and hence may still expose human subjects to risks. Nonetheless, compounds that turn out to be very toxic in LD50 tests at levels well below the necessary therapeutic levels are unlikely to be safe or worthwhile to test in humans. Whatever the rights and wrongs and limitations of pre-clinical toxicity testing, at present regulatory authorities require such testing on at least two species, one of which must be a non-rodent species such as the dog, before any human testing of a drug can begin.

Phase 1 trials

Having produced a candidate drug and completed the necessary pre-clinical testing package, the next step is testing in human subjects. Logically enough, this is termed a phase 1 trial. For many drugs, for example blood pressure pills, this testing will take place in 'normal', usually paid, volunteers. In general, these will be fit young men (not women, due to the risk of inadvertent damage to a foetus). For cancer drugs, which are often very toxic and frequently carcinogenic, this is clearly not an appropriate route, and phase 1 trials usually take place in patients who have exhausted standard treatment options. The classical phase 1 trial format is that the initial three patients are treated at a conservatively low dose and the effects observed. If no unacceptable toxicity occurs, then a further three patients will be treated at a higher dose, and so on. Clearly, for most drugs, eventually a dose level will be reached at which unacceptable side effects occur (termed 'dose-limiting toxicity', or DLT). If a patient experiences a DLT, additional patients are treated at the same dose level. If two or more out of six experience a DLT, then the 'maximum tolerated dose' (MTD) for the drug is reached and the trial ends. The dose level below the MTD will be used for further study.

The classical phase 1 trial has the merit of simplicity, but there are clearly limitations as well. Firstly, different patients will have varying susceptibility to potentially dose-limiting side effects. If the trial includes too many side-effect-prone patients, the estimated maximum tolerated dose will be too low, and vice versa. Secondly, not all drugs need to be used at the maximum tolerated dose. For example, a drug blocking a hormone receptor only needs to be given in sufficient quantity to block the target. Any additional drug given above this level is only adding toxicity with no benefit. For trials with drugs of this sort, it is therefore important to specify the endpoint required to avoid unnecessary drug exposure to participants.

The main problem with phase 1 trials relates to the needs of the patients. Mostly, these studies are happening in patients who have exhausted all standard therapy options and who are clearly desperate for further viable therapies. By its very nature, the phase 1 trial is mostly delivering drug below the likely therapeutic range with a consequent low chance of benefit. Furthermore, at least two of the last six patients entered in a study will receive too high a dose and will experience a high level of side effects. Finally, most drugs entering phase 1 will actually turn out to be of little therapeutic value due to either unforeseen problems preventing delivery of sufficient drug or simply a lack of efficacy against the target cancers. For most patients, therefore, entering a phase 1 trial needs to be seen largely as an act of altruism, and it is indeed true that many patients entering trials will say things like 'well if it helps people after me, it will be worth it'. Nonetheless, ethics committees and doctors must be careful to protect vulnerable and desperate patients from harm in these trials.

Phase 2

If an agent performs well in phase 1 – in other words, side effects are manageable and acceptable, usually with some evidence of a positive effect on the cancer, then a phase 2 trial will follow. The aim of phase 2 studies is to study the efficacy of the drug in more detail. The drug will be tested at the optimal dose defined in phase 1 in a group of patients assessed as likely to benefit from the drug. This is clearly different to phase 1 as the risk of under- or overdosing is much reduced, though it still remains, due to the limitations of the dose-finding mechanisms in phase 1 discussed above. Furthermore, as the patients are selected on the basis of likely benefit, the risk/benefit ratio for participants is much better. Typically, up to 40 or 50 patients will enter a phase 2 trial, and the endpoints will be efficacy, and of course safety, in the more defined, usually somewhat fitter, patient population.

Defining efficacy is a major problem. Generally, agents that produce tumour shrinkage are defined as active, and this has led to standardized ways of defining how much shrinkage constitutes a worthwhile response. The most widely used method is the RECIST (Response Evaluation Criteria In Solid Tumors) system, first published in 2000 and updated in January 2009. Disease responses are broadly classified as follows:

- complete response: all assessable disease disappeared;
- partial response: reduction in size by pre-specified amount of all assessable disease;
- stable disease: insufficient change to be put in another category;
- progressive disease: worsening of disease by pre-specified amount or appearance of new cancer deposits.

The principle underlying this system of assessment is simple; the application in practice is complex. As with many things, the devil is in the detail – the following is a list of tricky issues (not comprehensive) to illustrate the difficulties:

- How much should a tumour grow before it counts as progression?
- How much should it shrink to count as a response to treatment?
- What if some lumps shrink but not others?
- When should you carry out the response measurements (too early and you may under-report; too late and patients may have started relapsing)?

- How do you assess tumour deposits in tissues such as bone or pleura (the lining around the lung) where there is no discrete lump that can be measured?

This last point is a particular problem with certain diseases such as prostate cancer that mainly affect bone. Therefore, while response to treatment remains an important test of drug activity, a second set of measures based on how long a patient takes to start getting worse – termed the 'time to progression' – is increasingly used. This has proved particularly important with the new targeted molecular therapies for diseases like renal cancer. With this disease, large masses often shrink but by less than the standard RECIST criteria. On review of the scans in these patients, it became obvious that the tumours changed in appearance, with the centre appearing to be less 'active' than before – borne out when lumps were removed and found to have dead tissue in the middle. In parallel, tumour-related symptoms often improved. For these patients, therefore, prolonged 'stable' disease becomes a very worthwhile outcome. Improved time to progression is therefore frequently used as a means of assessing activity of an agent. Finally, of course, agents can be assessed for their effect on overall survival times. This is not frequently used in phase 2 as the principal outcome for a variety of reasons, mainly time – the aim is to establish as quickly as possible which agents to take forward for phase 3 licensing trials.

Phase 3 trials

If an agent shows encouraging activity in phase 2 with acceptable toxicity, it will then proceed into phase 3 trials in which the agent is compared to the current standard of care. Where the agent is a new drug, this will generally involve the drug company discussing the trial with the regulatory organizations such as the UK Medicines and Healthcare Regulatory Agency (MHRA), European Medicines Agency (EMA), and the US Food and Drug Administration (FDA). These bodies will have an opinion as to the appropriate comparator treatment and also the outcome required to obtain a licence. The comparator may be an existing drug or combination of drugs, or it may be what is termed 'best supportive care'. This latter option is chosen when there is no clear-cut standard therapy – patients receive whichever palliative measures the clinician thinks appropriate.

The hallmark feature of phase 3 trials is that the patients are randomly assigned between the treatment options. This ensures that patients will be evenly distributed between the various arms of the trial and minimizes the risk of differences in outcomes arising due to patients with a better or worse prognosis being concentrated in one arm of the trial. Whilst the design makes good scientific sense and is regarded as the 'gold standard' method of assessment, as always there are limitations.

Firstly and most obviously, where the control arm is best supportive care or worse still a placebo medication, there is understandable reluctance on the part of patients. Careful explanation and support is clearly required, particularly to make the point that if there is no other proven alternative, then treatment outside the trial will be no different to the control arm. Often, however, a phase 3 trial is not comparing the new drug with placebo but with the current standard therapy. This is generally a much easier discussion in the clinic as everyone receives treatment and the new medicine may be less good than the old one – we don't know until we do the trial. Even if the control is placebo, it is by no means a given that the new drug will turn out better – there are plenty of examples of trials in which the drug was no better than placebo, and even examples when the drug was worse – the drug was both toxic and ineffective.

Secondly, most new medicines will be only a little better than the existing ones, hence the likely differences between the trial arms will be small. In order to detect small differences, large sample sizes are necessary to ensure statistical confidence in the outcomes. Statistics is a much mocked, maligned, and misunderstood science, so it is helpful to illustrate why sample sizes need to be big with a simple example. Suppose we want to assess whether a coin used for a coin toss is evenly balanced or biased to either heads or tails. If we toss once, then we get either heads or tails (ignoring the possibility that the coin balances on its edge!). If we toss again and get the same, we have (say) 100% heads, 0% tails. No one would say the coin was biased on this size of sample, though. Suppose we carry on and get to 10 tosses – 6 heads, 4 tails – would we be confident that the coin was biased? Probably not. However, if we get to 100 tosses with 60 heads and 40 tails, or 1,000 tosses with 600 heads and 400 tails, we would have increasing confidence that the coin was indeed biased. The reverse of the problem is more difficult: if we got 501 versus 499, would we say the coin was biased? Again, probably not, but how about 510 versus 490? 520 versus 480? How similar can the numbers be in order that the difference is probably by chance rather than due to a biased coin? Even a big difference like 600 versus 400 can occur by chance with an unbiased coin, but would be very unlikely. The statistics plan for a trial is therefore key and will specify how many patients will be needed to reliably detect the minimum difference deemed to be clinically important in advance of the trial starting. For a trial testing a new drug in advanced cancer, this will be along the lines of an average improvement in survival of at least three months. As with our coin flip, this could arise by chance so the trial statistician will calculate how many patients are needed to show (or exclude) this difference reliably – usually defined (largely arbitrarily) as the chance result occurring fewer than 1 in 20 times.

For most modern trials, there will be a committee (usually called the Independent Data Monitoring Committee, IDMC, or Data and Safety Monitoring Committee, DSMC) set up to independently monitor the results as they accrue. This is in place to protect patients primarily – if there are unforeseen toxicity problems, for example, the trial may be stopped early. Later on in the trial, the IDMC can end the study if the predefined endpoints are met early.

This allows early dissemination of the data and allows other patients access to the drug earlier. Conversely, the IDMC can also determine that the trial is never likely to show significant differences and stop the trial early on grounds of futility.

Endpoints in trials are controversial. Trials are expensive, often $100 million plus, and hence drug companies want them to be as small and quick as possible. Conversely, regulators want the most reliable outcome measures and hence longer follow-up periods or larger sample sizes. Society at large has needs somewhere in between. We all want better medicines, and if we've got cancer, we want them now. Equally, we want them to be safe. Also, the larger and longer the trial, the more the drug company has to charge for the drug in order to pay back the higher development costs – see Chapter 5 for a more detailed discussion of this issue. As health budgets grow, so pressure to reduce drug costs rises, making availability of new drugs increasingly restricted for cancer patients in poorer economies. As a way out of these conflicting tensions, increasingly, researchers are looking for what are called 'surrogate' endpoints. The aim is to pick an early endpoint that will accurately predict the final outcome of the trial. The response rate in a phase 2 trial is an example of a surrogate endpoint used to select a drug for phase 3 study. The problem is that the correlation between response rate and the sort of endpoints regulators require, such as improved survival, is not sufficiently good to allow a high response rate in phase 2 to lead directly to a licence. The same will generally apply to comparisons of the response rates in randomized trials.

In order to get away from using survival-based comparisons, which clearly take a long time, investigators must show that some earlier measure reliably predicts the final outcome. An example of such a measure is the 'time to progression' mentioned above. This is the time taken for the tumour to grow or spread by pre-specified amounts and is commonly used as a registration trial endpoint in early breast cancer. In some disease settings, for example, PSA in prostate cancer, the candidate marker is unreliable, and drugs in prostate cancer are still currently stuck with needing to show improved survival to get a licence. In prostate cancer, studies are currently evaluating a novel method of response which is counting the number of circulating tumour cells. Typically, these are present in tiny numbers – around 5 per 7.5 millilitres of blood is the key cut-off level – a very tiny number of needles in a massive haystack of tens of millions of blood cells. If validated, such a test could greatly accelerate the pace of cancer drug development in diseases like prostate cancer currently stuck with overall survival endpoints. As shorter trials are cheaper, it could also reduce the price of the drug when licensed.

Comparisons of existing treatments

The phase 1–3 schema described above can broadly be fitted to any new technique or drug combination, however requirements differ in different countries. Trials comparing existing drugs in novel combinations are often undertaken by academic organizations such as Cancer Research UK or the US National Cancer Institute. Using the template above will give reliable results that can influence practice and are the gold standard for advancing medical practice in general. The system becomes much less clear with surgical techniques, radiotherapy equipment, other devices, and biomarkers, though. For example, new technologies such as robotic surgery are introduced as incremental improvements. These 'improvements' are treated as self-evident, when in fact they may be nothing of the sort. For example, comparing open with robot-assisted surgery: access routes to the body are different; the tactile connection between the surgeon's hands and the tissues is lost in robot-assisted surgery; control of bleeding or complications such as bowel perforation may present different risks, possibly requiring conversion from robot-assisted to an open conventional operation; theatre times may be longer when surgeons are training, and so on. It is clearly entirely plausible that each of these factors may substantially affect outcomes. In addition, there is the massive issue of cost. A surgical robot costs over £1 million, with another £100,000–£150,000 annual running costs. Even if the outcomes are better, how much is it worth paying for, say, earlier discharge from hospital?

One might expect that the introduction of such a technique, for example for prostate removal, would require the same sort of trials that new drugs for prostate cancer require, with equivalence or better in outcomes. No such trial has ever been carried out, yet surgical robots are working in major surgical centres across the world, particularly in the USA. Why the massive discrepancy? In essence, new devices simply have to demonstrate safety and fitness for the purpose for which they are designed. Where changes are genuinely small and incremental clearly a massive trial to show that a new scalpel is slightly better would be impractical and probably meaningless. At some point, the change ceases to be incremental and surgical robots seem to me to be a good example of this, yet are still treated as if they were simply a slightly better scalpel. In the USA in particular, buying a surgical robot has become an essential part of the marketing of a hospital – it is an iconic piece of kit – what go-ahead institution would want to be without one? Grappling with this issue is likely to become more and more important as healthcare systems struggle with rising costs. Conceivably, of course, new technologies may actually save costs. Sticking with the robots, it is not implausible that the claimed shorter learning curve, shorter hospital stay, and reduced complication rates could pay back the capital and running costs. At present, however, we simply don't know.

Similar arguments apply to tests such as imaging and other diagnostic tests. Again, there is an element of not needing to do research to validate the obvious – a scan with a sharper image is likely to be better than a fuzzy one! However, when we look more closely, things get more tricky. For example, one of the key drivers to decision-making is whether the cancer has spread to a particular organ. In general, if a scan looks abnormal in a particular area known to be at risk, it is likely that this represents disease. The

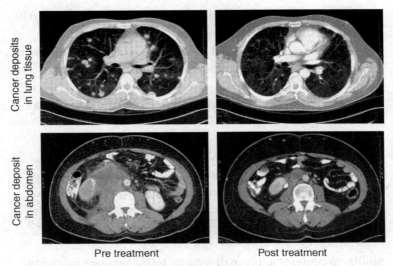

Cancer deposits in lung tissue

Cancer deposit in abdomen

Pre treatment   Post treatment

22. Examples of tumour responses on scans

converse is not the case, however – a negative scan could be negative or could mean the disease is below the threshold for detection. This is illustrated by the hypothetical liver scan discussed in Chapter 3. A good example of this sort of problem is the detection of cancer in lymph nodes. As lymph nodes are normal structures and cancer in lymph nodes is of similar density (and therefore imaging appearance) to the normal tissue, imaging can only tell us if nodes are of normal or abnormal dimensions – typically, the cut-off size is around 5 millimetres. Clearly, if we have a 4-millimetre cancer deposit replacing the bulk of a node, it will therefore look 'normal'.

Suppose a potentially better imaging test for node disease is developed, how should it be evaluated? Such a test would fall into the same sort of regulatory route as surgical devices – we need to show safety and fitness for purpose. Safety is straightforward – the phase 1/2 route clearly works fine, but how do we demonstrate 'fitness for purpose'? The answer is some form of clinical trial, but the question of endpoints is very tricky – how many 'normal' lymph nodes harbouring small cancers do we need to detect to be worthwhile? How many are we allowed to miss? How do we evaluate the 'true' positive and negative rates? Should we move to broader clinical outcomes rather than counting lymph nodes – for example, does the application of the test result in better clinical results, for example longer survival times, than the standard way of managing the patient?

These are all very difficult issues when applied to imaging technology when the acquisition costs of new scanners are very high. Even for technologies that augment existing scanners, for example new contrast medium drugs, the issues are substantial, and there is not a single consistent route across the globe.

Similar arguments apply to diagnostic tests. Again, at first sight, the problem would seem simple – if we have a blood test that correlates with the cancer, then we should use it as part of the basis for clinical decisions. However, if we examine the literature, we find many examples of tests that correlate with presence or absence of disease but very few are actually used clinically – why should this be? The principal answer to this is that the test has to give additional information over what we know already. For example, there are a whole range of urine tests that correlate with the presence of bladder cancer but none are used in the UK. Patients with suspected bladder cancer need a cystoscopy to confirm the diagnosis. The available urine tests are not reliable enough to exclude patients from a cystoscopy. Once the bladder has been examined, if a tumour is seen, a biopsy is needed. Again, the tests are not sufficiently reliable to obviate the need for biopsy. In addition, the excision biopsy is also part of the treatment, so however good the test, the patient still needs the operation. How about predicting prognosis? Again, the urine test is good but not as good as the pathological study of the removed tumour, so again it adds nothing. Given the above, the correct test for a diagnostic procedure is its effect on outcomes – can the test spare invasive procedures or predict which of a range of treatment options is best? This requires large-scale trials similar to those needed to license a drug and is the reason there are so few established tests or markers used in the clinic as decision aids.

There are examples of markers that correlate well with the disease and can be used to predict clinical events in advance of clinical symptoms or obvious scan changes. Examples of such markers include PSA in prostate cancer, CA125 in ovarian cancer, and AFP and HCG in testicular cancer. Even when good markers exist, they cannot necessarily replace other clinical methods of assessment. For example, while changes in PSA largely reflect changes in disease status, some treatments that affect the clinical outcomes (the bone-hardening drugs called bisphosphonates are a good example) have very little effect on PSA levels despite helping prevent bone damage by the cancer. Even more surprisingly, a recent huge study in ovarian cancer and the use of markers produced very counter-intuitive results. A rising level of CA125 in the blood accurately predicts clinical relapse. One might expect that treating relapse early would be better than waiting until symptoms developed. The study compared a policy of marker-driven treatment (that is, treatment for relapse started with rising marker levels) with clinical symptom-driven treatment. A total of around 1,500 women took part in the study, and the earlier introduction of treatment in women with more intensive monitoring did not affect survival times. Even more surprisingly, quality of life and anxiety levels were better in the women with the clinically driven treatment – tighter monitoring and earlier treatment were actually therefore inferior overall.

A huge focus of current research is individualized therapy – identifying markers that allow treatment to be tailored to the individual. There are many ways tumours can be characterized – by their DNA mutations, by their patterns of protein expression, by looking at the activities of different enzymes. However, while it is relatively easy to identify patterns that correlate with different outcomes, it will be obvious from the above discussion that this will not be sufficient to allow treatment to be altered. To demonstrate clinical value will require clinical trials comparing the candidate marker-driven policy with standard care. As the ovarian cancer example above shows, even having a good marker does not guarantee the expected result. A further problem that may emerge is that the numbers of candidate markers being developed may exceed the capacity of research teams to carry out trials, possibly many times over. Furthermore, markers effectively change a disease from being a homogenous entity to a number of distinct subentities. As good trials need large numbers, this makes doing trials more difficult – the disease effectively becomes rarer. This is illustrated by recent changes in renal cancer. A number of pathological variants had been described some time ago but until the advent of targeted small molecules, this made no difference to treatment options. As already discussed, the abnormalities in clear cell renal cancer (around 70% of the total) lead to new treatments. What then for the remaining 30%? Several different further subtypes make up this 30%, hence trials now become difficult as each is really rather uncommon. As a result, we don't really know how to manage these subgroups. These so-called 'orphan' diseases will become increasingly common and problematical as there will be little in the way of trial data to inform treatments, and trials will be difficult due to lack of numbers.

Conclusions

The coming years will see many exciting developments in new cancer drugs, new biomarkers, and exciting and futuristic technology such as surgical robots. How we incorporate these developments in practice will depend in large measure on clinical research to underpin their use. However, new technologies in particular will have a tendency to be introduced via the marketing rather than trials route. How we license, regulate, and fund these devices will become increasingly problematical as healthcare budgets come under pressure with an ageing population and the massive debt overhang of the credit crunch.

Chapter 5
The economics of cancer care

The previous chapters have illustrated the highly complex nature
of modern cancer care and the rapid rate of change in both
medical technology and drug therapy. These changes are underpinned by extensive investment in new treatments by both drug
and medical equipment manufacturers, as illustrated in the
previous chapter. Clearly, new treatments must be paid for and in
general will cost more than the older technologies they replace.
There are exceptions to this – for example, a treatment that
improved the cure rate could reduce downstream expenditure on
subsequent therapies and so may result in a net decrease in
healthcare resource use. Measuring these interdependent changes
is clearly complex, hence a lot of healthcare economic decision-
making is focused on the direct acquisition costs of the new
technology (which are easy to measure) rather than secondary
downstream changes. Frequently with cancer care, these costs are
focused near the end of life and result in contentious funding
dilemmas. How these dilemmas are dealt with by different
healthcare systems forms part of this chapter.

Economics also impinges on cancer care at a more macro-
economic level than the cost of an individual drug. In general,
the developed economies of the world have comprehensive
healthcare systems that broadly cover health issues from cradle

to grave. Different systems have different pros and cons, but the major difference is between the developed and less developed world. Clearly, if basic infrastructure is lacking, whether or not to buy an expensive new drug is not a relevant discussion for most of the population. It is possible to estimate the size of these effects: Figure 23 shows the interaction between per capita gross national product (pcGNP) and life expectancy in years. As can be seen, there are some countries with very low income and as would be expected, low life expectancy. However, there are others with pcGNP of less than $1,000 per year but where life expectancy exceeds 65 years. These countries include places like Egypt, Trinidad, and China. Common features of these countries are an integrated public health system and good perinatal care. Conversely, there are countries with pcGNP of more than $2,000 with life expectancy of less than 60 years. The problem here appears to be high levels of HIV infection. Thus in broad terms, how rich a country is will affect, not surprisingly, the quality of healthcare and life expectancy, but also other factors play an important part. Some of these factors can be readily influenced by factors within the control of governments – overall organization to get maximum impact from resources, public health campaigns, and so on. Conversely, at the upper end of the spectrum, once a certain level of national income is reached, there is very little further gain possible, with an apparent ceiling of life expectancy in the high 70s. Whether this will change in the future with improving technology remains to be seen.

If we move on to examine the effects of national income on cancer, we see another interesting effect. As wealth increases, so does the risk of developing cancer. This is partly an effect of lengthening life expectancy – if you don't starve or die young from infection, you have a much better chance of living to relative old age and getting cancer. Other factors are also at play: for example, once national income exceeds around $5,000 per person, cancer occurs at a rate of 250–400 cases per 100,000 people per year – see Figure 24. However, there are a number of countries with income

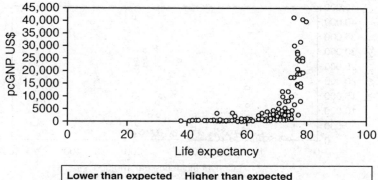

Lower than expected pcGNP$ >2000 Longevity <60	Higher than expected pcGNP$ <1000 Longevity >65
Namibia Botswana Gabon	Egypt, Trinidad, Honduras, Nicaragua, Vietnam, Mongolia, Indonesia, China, Surinam, Kyrgyzstan, Sri Lanka, Tajikistan, Turkmenistan, Uzbekistan, Armenia, Georgia, Azerbaijan, Albania, Macedonia, Solomon Islands

23. **National income per person and life expectancy**

in this bracket but with a cancer rate of less than one-third of this rate, all in the Middle East. This has been attributed to widespread adherence to more traditional, less Westernized lifestyles despite rising national income. Conversely, there is a cluster of countries with Western-style high cancer rates but income of less than $5,000 per head. These turn out to be former Soviet bloc states who seem at first glance to have the worst of outcomes – Western diseases at developing world incomes. On closer inspection, however, the picture is less gloomy – the low income is real but the high cancer rates reflect long life expectancy due to well-organized healthcare systems. The recent discussions about the relative merits of 'socialized medicine', and in particular the NHS and the US system, highlight the need for dispassionate analysis. Whilst it is true that there are differences in some outcomes between the US and UK, overall life expectancy is very

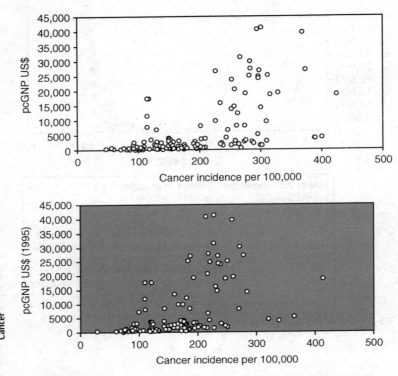

24. National income per person and cancer risk, for men (above) and for women (below)

similar for all countries with well-developed healthcare systems –
despite recent US Republican talk of NHS 'death panels', the truth
is that Western healthcare is pretty good at keeping most of its
citizens alive into old age.

Whilst all of this is true at the level of state funding, when cancer
therapy tends to hit the press is when access to a new therapy is
denied someone, usually presented as a variant of the staple news
story of 'patient refused life-saving drug by faceless bureaucrat'.
This is the origin of the Republican allegations about NHS death

panels (in truth, of course, US patients with no healthcare will also be denied the same treatment by a different set of bureaucrats or perhaps their bank manager). Why do these stories occur in some of the wealthiest countries in the world? What are the likely future trends in funding and costs?

Like most commodities, medical care tends to cost more year on year – inflation. It is possible to measure the rate of medical inflation, and in general this turns out to be higher than the underlying inflation rate in the economy. This is important as it means that without cost-cutting, healthcare over time will consume a bigger proportion of national income in keeping up with new technologies. This is best illustrated by the US economy where the medical inflation rate in 2008 was 6.9% – roughly double the rest of the economy. On current projections, this would see the US health spend increase from 17% of national income in 2008 to 20% by 2017. The massive changes in the world economy since the banking crisis make it very unlikely that this can be sustained. Similar figures apply in all the major economies. Why are costs rising in this fashion? After all, when the NHS was set up, Aneurin Bevin, one of its key architects, envisaged falling costs with time as health improved. The reason lies in the costs of developing new treatments. A licensing trial for a cancer treatment will typically cost around £100,000,000. Newly licensed drugs thus need to recoup these massive development costs, plus the costs of all the drugs that fell by the wayside in the process and will thus never generate any revenue. Patent life remaining by the time a drug is licensed is typically 10 years or less, as drugs need to be patent-protected many years before the licensing process is complete. The bulk of the cost of a new drug therefore reflects the costs incurred before licence – the actual manufacturing, while expensive, is typically only a small proportion of the price per pill. When a drug comes off patent the cost of a drug will usually fall with generic competition by around 90–95%, reflecting this.

The price charged for a new drug will thus be geared to paying back the massive development costs and then turning a profit before the patent licence expires. With globalization, prices tend to be similar worldwide, making new drugs particularly hard to afford in poorer countries. The pricing policies of pharmaceutical companies are not in the public domain but are presumably set to maximize income worldwide. For some countries, such as the UK, Australia, and New Zealand, this will often be above the price the health system is prepared to pay. This is presumably offset by the higher income generated by the greater price obtained in less restrictive health systems. For example, in France, once a drug is licensed, it can be freely prescribed by the relevant specialist with no direct expenditure cap. This has a big influence on rates of uptake and total spend, as we shall see later in the chapter. However, the ongoing trends of medical inflation and rising costs of development will exert pressure on the budgets everywhere and make access to therapies more and more of a problem. Similar arguments apply to devices – see, for example, the new robotic surgical technology described in the previous chapter.

A recent report from the well-respected Karolinska Institute in Helsinki examined the issue of cancer drug funding in some detail. The report examined the trends across the European Union and compares spending patterns in different member countries as well as summarizing worldwide issues. Globally, the cancer drugs market was valued at $34 billion in 2006, rising to $43 billion by 2008, with an annual research spend of $6–$8 billion by the pharmaceutical industry and a further $3.6 billion by the US National Cancer Institute and €1.4 billion in the EU. Around half of all the drugs in trials worldwide are cancer therapies. Within the EU, sales of cancer drugs per 100,000 population increased from less than €500,000 in 1996 to more than €2.5 million by 2007 – a six-fold increase in 10 years. Furthermore, this rise was not driven by expensive new drugs, though these are a growing strain on budgets, but mostly by increasing use of existing drugs. These two trends are illustrated in Figure 25, which shows the

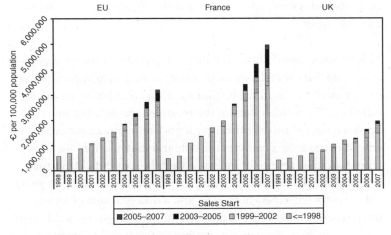

25. Sales of cancer drugs 1998–2007 in the EU

increase in drug spending broken down by the year in which a drug was licensed. The figure also shows the contrast between spending in France, where there are essentially few controls on oncology prescribing, and the UK, where it is tightly regulated.

Why should older drugs have seen such a big increase in expenditure? The answer lies in how drugs are licensed and then subsequently used. If we look at figure 18 in Chapter 3 to illustrate the breakdown of cancer therapy, we can see that around 40% of patients develop advanced cancer at some stage, most of whom will ultimately die from the disease. New drugs are generally tested initially in this group of ultimately incurable patients with limited options. In breast cancer, for example, only a minority of patients die from the disease and hence expenditure on a newly licensed, end-stage drug will be relatively limited. However, if a drug works well in this group, it will often work better in earlier patients with potentially curable disease at high risk of relapse after their initial therapy. This group makes up around half of the patients who end up with advanced disease. Trials of successful end-stage drugs will thus take place in these patients and if successful the drug will 'migrate' into the earlier disease group.

This process is well illustrated by the Herceptin (trastuzumab) story. The drug was shown to prolong survival in advanced breast cancer in 2002. From the beginning, Herceptin has attracted huge publicity. The novel nature of the treatment rapidly became known amongst breast cancer patients leading to a clamour to enter the trials. So great was the demand that a lottery for trial entry had to be set up for interested eligible patients. After the drug obtained a licence, its high price (around £30,000 per year) led to restricted access in the UK and a different sort of lottery – the post-code lottery of UK cancer funding – began for a different group of women. The subsequent highly vocal campaign by women successfully overturned the restrictions but also set a precedent for other groups seeking access to expensive therapies that still bedevils purchasing authorities in the UK in particular.

Subsequent trials in earlier disease showed in 2006 that if given to women with early high-risk disease after surgery, Herceptin reduced the chances of a disease recurrence by about half compared to previous therapies. The licence for Herceptin was thus extended to this earlier disease group the same year. Unfortunately, we cannot currently identify those who will relapse after surgery and radiotherapy. As most women in the early, high-risk group were already cured by standard therapy, the numbers eligible to receive the drug increased hugely (about four-fold in the UK) – all patients at risk have to be treated, not just those destined to relapse. Following a vocal campaign by women with the disease, the drug was made available on the NHS to all eligible patients.

How, therefore, do healthcare systems make decisions about new treatments? Suppose a new treatment costs £30,000 and improves survival by 6 months, from 12 to 18 months. What is the real cost of providing this treatment?

- £30,000
- £30,000 minus the treatment it replaces
- £30,000 minus the treatment it replaces and minus any consequent savings in other supportive care

There is no correct answer – it depends on who is paying for what. Answer 1 is the cost to the patient if the treatment is not reimbursed by the healthcare system. This is sometimes the case in the UK where the NHS sets limits on which drugs it will buy. The old standard of care will be covered but not the new drug. Increasingly, it is also a problem for patients in insurance-based systems where the extra drug falls outside the reimbursement package covered by the insurance. Answer 2 is the price to a hospital providing specialist care where the hospital budget per patient is fixed (as happens in hospitals in the NHS and some managed-care systems in the USA). Answer 3 is the price to the organization funding the totality of the patient's care: this may be the state via structures like the NHS or an insurance company. This then raises the further question of what exactly is included in the associated costs. For example, terminal care costs will probably be similar whenever a patient dies. However, if the survival time is longer, as in the example, they may then fall in a different financial year to the drug costs – how long must costs be deferred to count as savings? This is particularly the case with treatments which increase the cure rate, for which such costs may be postponed for many years. Again, there is no single simple answer to such questions – different healthcare systems tend to resolve these dilemmas in different ways. It is worth examining the sort of methodologies used by public health specialists and insurance companies in making these decisions on whether to fund a particular treatment.

A frequently used method is to estimate the cost per year of extra life generated by the new treatment. A correction for the overall quality of that life is often also applied. The aim is to produce a measure known as a quality adjusted life year (QALY). For example, a treatment that prolonged your life by a year but at a 50% reduction in quality would be costed as 0.5 QALY. This sounds very neat, and it allows purchasers of healthcare to compare a drug therapy that prolongs life by 3 months with a hip replacement which improves quality of life with no effect on life expectancy. For well-established treatments such as surgery and radiotherapy, patients are frequently cured, and thus this cost is spread over a large number of life years gained. Thus, although major surgery is expensive, it has a very low cost per QALY in most cases. In contrast, new drugs that prolong survival by relatively modest amounts in end-stage disease often have a very high cost/QALY, and this is where the problems start, as will be illustrated below.

An immediate problem with adjusting for quality of life is clearly apparent – how do we define how much a person's quality of life is affected? For example, Mr A leads a sedentary life and mainly enjoys watching TV for recreation, therefore an impairment which stops him running will matter very little. Mr B, however, is a keen triathlete and finds the same loss of mobility hugely distressing. Clearly, any quality adjustment is subjective and will depend on those affected. Somehow an average value must be arrived at and added to the equation.

A second problem is how to measure the gain in survival. This may seem straightforward, but often licensing trials will focus on the time taken for the disease to worsen (so-called 'time to progression' – see Chapter 4) rather than overall survival. Subsequent 'salvage' treatment may therefore improve the outcomes of the patients in the initial control arm of the trial. Endpoints for these trials are set by the regulatory authorities, such as the US Food and Drug Administration and the European Medicines Agency, and determine whether a company is granted a licence to market their product. However, just because a drug can be marketed does not mean that a healthcare system will buy it.

In order to illustrate how this process works, I will run through the recent trials carried out with a new drug in advanced kidney cancer. In the trial, patients on the placebo were deteriorating twice as quickly as those on the new drug called sorafenib. The Independent Data Monitoring Committee for the trial decided the study should be stopped on ethical grounds and all the placebo patients still alive were offered the new drug. When the overall survival times were subsequently analysed, the patients initially on the new drug lived longer than those on placebo. However, due to the salvage effect from the crossover from placebo to active drug, the survival advantage for the new drug was much smaller than would have been expected from the effect on time to progression. It is thus impossible to calculate the survival benefit of sorafenib in advanced kidney cancer as this trial can never be ethically repeated with a no-treatment arm. Any estimates for the cost per QALY for this disease are thus doubly flawed – the effect on quality of life is subjective and the true survival gain unknown. This double uncertainty paralysed the UK decision-making process for kidney cancer from 2006 to 2009.

The use of decision-making based on quality-adjusted survival has been pioneered extensively by a UK body with the somewhat Orwellian title of National Institute for Health and Clinical Excellence, usually known as NICE. This body seeks to advise the health service which treatments it should purchase on behalf of the patients and which treatments are not considered good value for money and should not be routinely funded. NICE does not consider unlicensed or experimental treatments. Some other European countries have adopted similar methodologies, but as yet the more free-market approach in the USA has shied away from such central direction. NICE will often take months or even years from the initial licence to give an opinion on a drug. In the UK, the NHS funding is split between 'purchasers' and 'providers'. Currently, the purchasers are called Primary Care Trusts (PCTs) and are tasked with making the same decisions (to buy or not to buy a particular treatment) on a local basis. At the time of writing, in 2011, this purchaser role is set to be transferred to family doctors (GPs) under forthcoming NHS reforms. The current PCTs discharge this role with varying degrees of competence and thoroughness, often simply providing the cheapest option until forced to provide a more expensive one by subsequent NICE guidance. This leads in turn to the (in)famous UK post-code lottery – as PCTs are geographically based, access to any NHS treatment is determined by the patient's address and the local PCT decision-making process. In 2008, this resulted in the highest spending PCTs allocating around £15,000 per patient for cancer care compared to around £5,000 for the lowest spending ones. In my own clinic, patients with a Birmingham post-code (a high-spend area) enjoy good access to, for example, the latest kidney cancer drugs. Conversely, most of the surrounding counties have relatively low cancer drug spends and access to the same drugs is severely restricted. As patients clearly talk to each other in the waiting room the level of frustration and anger generated can be readily imagined. We carried out an audit of survival times by post-code for our patients with advanced kidney cancer. Patients from the low-spend areas survived around 7–8 months on average, compared to around 2 years for those from the higher spending Birmingham area – a very real and worthwhile difference. In addition, patients denied access to the expensive drugs had roughly three times as many visits to hospital due to increased rates of disease complications from their untreated cancer. This state of affairs persisted for 3 years from 2006 (when the new kidney cancer drugs were first licensed) to early 2009 when NICE finally recommended that one of these drugs, sunitinib, be made available to all kidney cancer patients (though access to other recently licensed kidney cancer drugs remains heavily restricted). Clearly, the PCTs not funding these drugs would argue that they have used this money elsewhere to produce a bigger gain for a different group of patients. I am not aware, however, that there is any good evidence that poorer outcomes occur in other groups of Birmingham patients compared to their shire county neighbours as a result of lack of funds. The present UK system strikes me therefore as cumbersome, unnecessarily bureaucratic, and in many cases ill-informed. Those making the decisions, allegedly on behalf of the public, are not in any way publicly accountable for their decisions – they are not elected, for example – and often will not publicly defend them. On the other hand, in an era of rising costs, an ageing population, and shrinking budgets some form of choice must be made and thus structures like NICE will probably become more common worldwide in the future.

The proposed new UK purchasing arrangements will mean that one group, GPs, will be both purchasers and providers, with a second group, the specialist care sector in hospitals, being purely providers. It will mean GP consortia will have a financial vested interest in keeping patients out of hospitals, which may or may not be a good thing. On the other hand, they will have to justify to their own patients, in a way that the current PCTs do not, why they have chosen to refuse funding for certain treatments, as inevitably they must. It remains to be seen whether the possibility of lower management costs translates, as the government hopes, into better frontline care, as it is not immediately clear to me why GPs are the best people to decide on specialist care choices.

The cumbersome decision-making process in the UK also tends to delay uptake of new cancer drugs and reduce overall spending compared to other similar European economies. Although not formally published, it is estimated that NICE has a target spend of up to £30,000 per quality-adjusted life year gained, treatments costing more being denied funding. Other countries have less formalized methods, but appear to informally apply higher cut-off levels. Currently, the UK spends around 60% of the levels reached in countries such as France and Germany on cancer drugs as a result of this lower cut-off point. This difference seems to be particularly focused on cancer therapy as no such disparity exists in other specialisms such as cardiovascular disease or psychiatry, two other big-spend areas. This is well illustrated by the patterns of spending on sunitinib in kidney cancer since licence in 2006, with

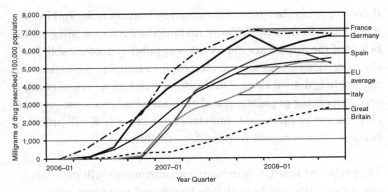

26. Usage of the drug sunitinib in the EU

the UK showing a late, slow rise in spending on the drug compared to the EU average and Italy, France, Germany, and Spain in particular (Figure 26). It cannot be a coincidence that the relatively poor cancer outcomes seen in the UK compared to our European neighbours occur in a country with a relatively low spend on cancer drugs and big disparities in spend per patient by post-code.

The future trends in spending also look challenging. There are currently 77 drugs licensed in the UK for the treatment of cancer (this ignores drugs for supportive care). Around 25 of these were licensed 1995–2005. There are an estimated 50 drugs seeking approval in the period 2007–12. Clearly, not all of these drugs will succeed in jumping the final hurdle. Furthermore, many will offer only very small gains over alternative treatment options. Some of these drugs, possibly many, will, however, offer big further gains. In addition, there will be the ongoing trend of existing new expensive drugs migrating to earlier disease settings and larger markets as illustrated for Herceptin in breast cancer. All of this will undoubtedly put further heavy financial pressure on all health economies. An interesting trend at the international conferences I attend has been discussion of these points. Until recently, this was only a topic of interest in the UK due to our relatively poor access to new drugs. Increasingly, even US speakers, with previously apparently bottomless health budgets to draw upon, have started to discuss affordability of new therapies. The healthcare reform package of Barack Obama has also put this same issue solidly on the mainstream political agenda in the USA.

There are a few trends potentially relieving pressure. Firstly, older drugs when they come off patent usually plummet in price, often by up to 95%. Secondly, if the improvement in outcome is large enough, there may be compensatory savings in other health costs, though the expenditure is now and the savings are later and may be hard to trace (and may even accrue to another healthcare provider). Thirdly, better predictors of disease behaviour may allow us to target our expensive therapies on those most likely to benefit. For example, if we knew which breast cancer patients would be cured by surgery alone (the majority), we could save a huge proportion of our adjuvant therapy drug costs. Research into such predictive biomarkers is one of the hottest areas in cancer at present for this reason. Research into new clinical trials methodologies may also help to reduce development times and thereby drug costs.

Conclusions

How these factors play out in the coming years remains to be seen, and it is likely that different solutions will emerge across the globe. Within Europe, we are likely to see the principle of universal coverage for state-of-the-art care increasingly slipping. The picture in the UK where NICE decides on affordability is likely to become more widespread as a model for decision-making, despite the problems experienced by NICE operationally. This then raises the linked issue of top-up funding, already a political hot potato in the UK. Private insurance to top up state provision may also become more the norm as the costs are much lower than for policies aimed at replacing state provision. In the USA, a major issue of partial coverage remains. Even for those with insurance, I suspect we will begin to see some attempt to limit expenditure on the most expensive cancer therapies. Outside the major Western economies, we are likely to see cancer incidence rising as life expectancy improves with economic growth. As seen in this chapter and the previous one, the best-value cancer therapies are surgery and radiotherapy, and we are likely to see a growth in these services in developing economies. The extra gain from drug therapies is relatively small, so access to these is likely to be more restricted to cheaper, older drugs, with the most expensive therapies confined to a small minority in these countries.

Chapter 6

Alternative and complementary approaches to cancer care

Research shows that at least half of cancer patients use complementary or alternative medicines in addition to conventional medicine (and one suspects that a lot of the remainder are simply not telling us). These come in many varieties and include traditional therapies used by patients from ethnic minorities. Although the terms 'complementary' and 'alternative' are sometimes used interchangeably, it is helpful to distinguish between different varieties of what may be termed to be outside mainstream medical practice. I will therefore refer to complementary medicines as those aimed at running alongside conventional therapies as a form of support. An example would be aromatherapy, which does not fundamentally conflict with the patient continuing their conventional therapy. Indeed, aromatherapy may aid compliance with treatment or reduce the need for additional medications such as laxatives or painkillers. As well as quasi-medical therapies like aromatherapy, there are treatments such as acupuncture and homeopathy that may be available both via mainstream healthcare and via other 'therapists'. Alternative medicines, on the other hand, are aimed at replacing the mainstream treatment with one that conventional medicine would regard as unproven at best and harmful at worst. In practice, it is impossible to rigidly separate treatments into one or other category, as while one patient may use a remedy alongside the conventional, another may use the same remedy in place of it – the distinction is one of intent as much as content.

There are a huge number of different alternative and complementary medicines, including homeopathy, acupuncture, dietary therapies, herbal remedies, aromatherapy, as well as techniques such as crystal therapy, visualization, and traditional therapies used by ethnic minorities. A full analysis of each of these is beyond the scope of this book, so I will try and select a few examples to make general points about how complementary and alternative treatments interact with cancer therapy. Before doing so, it is worth getting a feel for the massive extent of usage of such treatments. While countries may vary, usage in the USA is likely to be pretty typical of use in the developed world. As it is easy to quantify spending in the USA, I will give a breakdown of recent figures produced by the American National Institutes for Health. The headline figure is that 88 million Americans spent $33.9 *billion* on complementary or alternative medicines in 2007. This amounted to over 10% of all 'out of pocket' expenditure on health in the USA. In addition, a further $23 billion was spent on vitamin and mineral supplements. Given the very high medical bills faced by US citizens, it is clearly astonishing that they would spend such a sum in addition. At the 2007 exchange rate, this would have provided all healthcare for the UK population for about 6 months. These figures clearly relate to total expenditure, not money spent specifically by cancer patients; however, they do give a good feel for the extent to which these treatments are used. Similar expenditures occur in all industrialized countries. Why do citizens in all the most educated societies in the world, generally provided with healthcare which, as we have seen, keeps most of them alive into old age, shell out such huge sums on additional, mostly unproven, therapies? Clearly, in less wealthy societies, traditional remedies may be all that part of the population can afford, and thus different forces may be at play.

Before moving on to try and address this, it is worth looking at a breakdown of what the money goes on. Again, I will refer to the US figures, and clearly the split elsewhere may vary, but I believe it gives a feel of the sorts of things people want. If we understand that, it may help explain the paradox above.

The biggest category in the US report is described as 'non-vitamin, non-mineral natural products'. These are presumably herbal remedies of various sorts – as already noted, this *excludes* the expenditure of around $23 billion on vitamin supplements and minerals such as selenium. A further $4.1 billion is spent on techniques that focus on mental wellbeing with or without a component of exercise – yoga, for example. Clearly, it is debatable whether these really belong here as the individual's motivation is clear – it makes them feel good. As this clearly is a benefit in itself, I do not think further discussion is necessary. The same applies to the $0.2 billion spent on relaxation techniques.

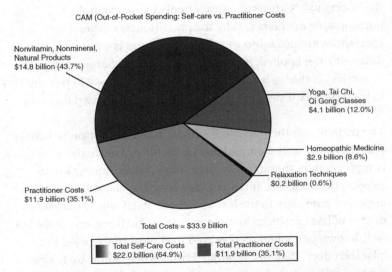

CAM (Out-of-Pocket Spending: Self-care vs. Practitioner Costs

Nonvitamin, Nonmineral, Natural Products
$14.8 billion (43.7%)

Yoga, Tai Chi, Qi Gong Classes
$4.1 billion (12.0%)

Homeopathic Medicine
$2.9 billion (8.6%)

Relaxation Techniques
$0.2 billion (0.6%)

Practitioner Costs
$11.9 billion (35.1%)

Total Costs = $33.9 billion

| Total Self-Care Costs $22.0 billion (64.9%) | Total Practitioner Costs $11.9 billion (35.1%) |

27. Expenditure on complementary and alternative medicines in the USA, 2007

Most of the remainder is either grouped as practitioner costs ($11.9 billion) or homeopathic medicine $2.9 billion (it's not clear whether this reflects the 'medicines' themselves or the total cost including practitioner fees). Either way, this is an astonishing sum to have been spent in a society as litigious as the USA. For a practitioner of conventional medicine, the route to a licence is long and heavily policed. Any licensed drug will have been through stringent approval procedures to demonstrate efficacy, safety, and fitness for purpose. Thus both the practitioner and products used are heavily regulated. Step outside the rules and stringent penalties apply both to practitioners and sellers of medicines and devices. Failure of either to perform to the expected standard will result in legal and often financial penalties. In conventional medicine, a drug company cannot legally sell a treatment for, say, asthma without evidence that it works a reasonable amount of the time.

For most alternative and complementary medicines, no such tests apply in most countries. Regulation is either absent or internal to the 'speciality'. No tests of efficacy apply to, for example, homeopathic medicines. Why the practitioners of these specialities are not subject to these basic rules is a mystery. Even if different rules applied, in other walks of life to charge for a good or service on the basis that it has certain properties will be subject to legal penalty if the item does not fulfil the advertised function.

The truth is that the purveyors of these remedies appear to believe that they work and their patients do likewise. Alternative and complementary therapies are therefore in reality more akin to religion than science, and this goes a long way to explaining their apparent immunity to the law, as religion itself enjoys the same degree of legal privilege in most countries. Furthermore, there is a well-known phenomenon observed in clinical trials called the 'placebo effect'. Patients in blinded trials where some are taking dummy pills called placebos will often experience the beneficial effects (and bizarrely, sometimes the minor side effects) expected from the active drug. This effect is often substantial and is in many ways highly desirable – there is clearly no risk of serious drug-related adverse events. The body is healing itself. Clearly, therefore, if the alternative 'practitioner' and the patient collude in a belief that a treatment works, it often will. Does this mean it is an honest practice? In my opinion, it does not – I believe these remedies should be subject to the same tests of efficacy as any other product, whether medicinal or not.

Furthermore, it is not the case that no harm is done by an ineffective product – it depends on how it alters the treatment of the patient. Clearly, if, say, homeopathy is used for a minor, self-limiting condition such as soft tissue injury, then no long-term harm is likely. If it is used in place of a standard therapy for cancer, AIDS, or tuberculosis (as some of its proponents advocate), then clearly deterioration can occur while the patient is forgoing some more effective therapy.

As already discussed, the gold standard way to assess any medicine, conventional or otherwise, is in a controlled trial. These are widely used to assess conventional medicines but have also been used to test complementary or alternative medicines such as homeopathic remedies as well as with techniques like acupuncture (where the control is sham acupuncture – a needle is inserted but in the 'wrong' place).

The basis of homeopathy is that 'like cures like'. Practitioners take compounds that induce a symptom, say, nausea, and then dilute the active compounds sequentially to the point when not a single molecule of the original substance remains. Proponents claim that the 'potentizing' involved in making a homeopathic remedy somehow 'imprints' the water molecules with properties that will have medicinal effects. The effects are generally held to be the reverse of the symptom induced by the agent the homeopathic pharmacy began with – hence the medicine from the example above would be used to treat nausea. For such a therapy to be effective would require a reworking of a substantial body of physics, chemistry, and tissue biology, all of which is currently lacking. Even if we concede that our knowledge of these disciplines is imperfect, it is not unreasonable to expect that there would be evidence from clinical trials of effectiveness. If there were convincing trial evidence of efficacy, clearly the underlying scientific orthodoxy would need to be re-examined to accommodate the new evidence. We therefore need to examine the clinical trial evidence for homeopathy.

A number of controlled trials with homeopathy have indeed been carried out. In 2005, the respected medical journal *The Lancet* published an article analysing the results from 110 trials of homeopathy that included a placebo. These trials were compared with 110 similar trials of conventional medicine (referred to in the homeopathy literature as allopathy, meaning 'other than the disease'). The *Lancet* article concluded there was no evidence of a coherent effect from homeopathy that could not be explained by the placebo effect. In contrast, the conventional trials were able to show effects from conventional medicines over and above the placebo in similar conditions. Homeopathy would thus seem to sit solidly in the 'alternative' category as its practitioners promote it as exactly that, an alternative to conventional medicine. With no evidence of solid benefit, this seems an irresponsible view to take, especially as homeopathy is promoted for use in all manner of diseases including potentially lethal conditions such as asthma, tuberculosis, and AIDS. This view is endorsed by bodies such as the World Health Organization (WHO) which recently issued a warning stating that the use of homeopathy to treat conditions such as tuberculosis and malaria was dangerous, and it said quite categorically that lives were being lost as a result. Hence on every level, when the 'science' of homeopathy is examined, it clearly poses problems by the yardsticks of conventional science – there is no coherent physical basis for its mode of action, nor convincing trial evidence of efficacy. Despite this lack of evidence, homeopathy is available on the NHS in the UK, and millions worldwide, including the Prince of Wales, believe in its effectiveness.

So why do so many patients use these treatments? Most people have only the most sketchy understanding of science and tend to view the claims of scientists and alternative practitioners as equally valid alternatives. This view is peculiarly limited to biology – no one wants to use 'alternative' approaches to, for example, engineering or piloting an aeroplane; they stick with the laws of aerodynamics and trained pilots. I believe that in many, if not most, cases, people are simply desperate and want to hedge their bets by backing both horses. Patients who have run out of curative conventional options often pursue these therapies and are clearly vulnerable to exploitation. Extreme varieties of these treatments often require the patient to travel to countries where regulation of such therapies is less strict than it is within, say, the USA or European Union.

Patients also frequently adopt unusual dietary approaches. Often, the underlying rationale, if there is one, will mix cause and effect. The logic underpinning these diets often runs something like this: the risk of getting a number of cancers may be increased by a lack of X in the diet (possible), therefore taking X will restore balance and treat the cancer. This leads to patients taking, for example, vitamin or mineral supplements. As a proposal, this is at least testable – we can do a trial with the supplement in question and see whether it impacts on the outcomes experienced by patients. Another common theme in anticancer diets is to pick a particular component of the diet, such as animal fat – the underlying logic being that a number of common cancers have been linked to an excess of animal fats in the diet, therefore giving up animal fats will treat the cancer (unlikely). Substituting the word 'smoking' for 'animal fats' in lung cancer illustrates the futility of this – if all you had to do to treat lung cancer was stop smoking, far fewer would die from it. Sadly, stopping smoking has very little impact on the grimly predictable outcome of most lung cancer. Similarly, evidence that these sorts of 'subtraction' diets impact cancer survival is also conspicuous by its absence. Another more recent example I have observed in patients turning up in my clinics is the claim that eating sugar is bad, as this 'fuels' the cancer. As all complex carbohydrates are digested down to sugars in the gut before being absorbed, this is highly unlikely to be a good therapy, especially as organs such as the liver and pancreas very tightly regulate sugar levels in the blood.

Despite the flawed logic and lack of evidence, patients will often adopt new diets in response to a diagnosis of cancer, frequently giving up foods enjoyed for decades to adopt a diet with alleged 'detoxification' or 'healing' properties, or adding supplements to 'boost' the body's defence mechanisms. At the extremes, both practitioners and adherents often promote these approaches with a fervour approaching the religious. Indeed, adherence to these doctrines in many ways parallels religious observance, with denial and self-sacrifice being potentially rewarded by improved wellbeing. Like religious observance, direct evidence of efficacy is not required – belief that it works is sufficient. Furthermore, failure of the technique to work can be interpreted as an indication of insufficient diligence in the application of the regime rather than an indication of lack of efficacy.

In 1990, a team of three of us (two oncologists and a psychiatrist) visited the Gerson Centre in Tijuana in Mexico. The Gerson plan is based on a curious mix of a 'detoxifying' diet (vegan, crushed fruit and vegetable juices, no added salt) and the frankly odd (regular fresh coffee enemas). Dr Max Gerson developed the diet to treat various ailments, including diabetes (he treated Albert Schweitzer) and tuberculosis. Ironically, he was driven from the USA for advocating the diet for diabetes, at the time treated with a high-fat, low-carbohydrate diet. It subsequently turned out that the 'Gerson' high-fibre, low-fat diet actually was a good treatment for diabetes, but this was only realized many years later. This does demonstrate the need to evaluate therapies in a scientific way – when this was done, it proved the value of low-fat, high-carbohydrate diets for diabetes. However, after being expelled from the USA, Gerson continued to advocate the therapy for a range of other conditions, including cancer, heart disease, and arthritis. The US National Cancer Institute carried out investigations in 1947 and 1959 to assess whether the Gerson regime had any effect on cancer outcomes, concluding both times that there was no convincing evidence of a treatment effect. Our own review of cases selected by the Centre in 1990 came to the same conclusion, which we published in the medical journal *The Lancet*. Patients at the centre undoubtedly believed they were benefiting, and in a sense, for the reasons outlined above, they were getting spin-off psychological benefits from feeling more in control of their fate. There is a flip-side to this, however, in that patients who invest a lot of energy and belief in such treatments inevitably feel that they have somehow failed when their disease worsens. This is often painful in itself, but can sometimes drive them to more extreme adherence to a regime in the mistaken belief that, if only they could adhere more perfectly, then improvement would follow.

There is a further problem with some dietary approaches like Gerson therapy. Whilst in some ways the diet (at least, without the coffee enemas) could be regarded as healthy, it may be unsuited to some types of cancer patients. For example, patients with pancreatic cancer tend to lose weight rapidly. Following a diet that will tend to bring about weight loss in healthy individuals is thus actively harmful when weight loss is part of the problem being faced. Also, as already noted, many patients tend to 'mix and match' the conventional with the alternative. Treatments such as chemotherapy can lead to digestive problems and promote weight loss. It is thus easy to see that a very high-fibre diet, relatively low in calories, may not be ideal in such circumstances. The alternative practitioner would, of course, argue that the problem here is the conventional not the alternative part of the treatment. This would be an acceptable line to run if these treatments were subject to proper scrutiny with proven efficacy. For Gerson therapy, despite 90 years of use, many published case reports, and reviews by academics, there is still not a single published clinical trial. Rather as with drugs, I feel it is for the proponents of such treatments to arrange trials, just as the drug companies have to demonstrate effectiveness to obtain a licence for their products. There may well be patients who do benefit from 'alternative' dietary approaches, but at present the evidence is lacking.

Closely linked to alterations in diet are nutritional supplements based on either vitamins and minerals or herbal mixtures (sometimes called 'nutriceuticals'). These therapies are potentially more amenable to conventional clinical evaluation than the complete lifestyle change advocated by groups such as the Gerson therapists. The simplest version of dietary supplementation is with either vitamins or minerals. Vitamins (a derivative of the compound words 'vital amines') are chemicals present in tiny amounts in foodstuffs and are essential for the body to maintain normal functions. A good example is vitamin C, derived from various fruits, particularly citrus ones. Shortage of vitamin C leads to that scourge of ancient mariners, scurvy, a condition in which wound healing is impaired, tissues become fragile and bruise and bleed easily, gums bleed, and teeth fall out – the body's so-called 'connective tissue' fails to connect things properly. Clearly, therefore, vitamin C is essential for life, but if we have sufficient, is there any benefit in taking more? The Nobel prizewinner Linus Pauling became convinced that there was benefit in so-called 'mega-doses' of the vitamin, and he vigorously advocated the practice for various ailments from the common cold to cancer (it should be noted that he got the Nobel for physics not medicine). Now here we have a readily testable hypothesis – vitamin C can be put in tablets and assessed like any other medicine. This was duly done in various settings and the answer was a resoundingly negative one – dietary supplementation of vitamin C above normal levels did not help fight cancer (or anything else). Nonetheless, hard evidence of lack of efficacy in no way prevents the alternative practitioners from continuing to promote the use of the agent, as the most cursory of online searches will confirm.

Even doing trials with simpler substances – minerals – turns out to be very difficult. For example, selenium is present in vegetables and is an essential component of tissues, being involved in the maintenance of the integrity of epithelial membranes – the lining cells of the body's various tubes and glands. It is these cells that give rise to the common cancers, and thus a lack of selenium would seem a potential candidate for a dietary top-up. Further studies demonstrated that populations with lower selenium levels had a higher risk of cancer. This prompted trials of selenium supplementation in patients with cancer, and one famous study in skin cancer showed that the patients receiving the extra selenium had a lower risk of getting a second cancer – of the prostate. The problem was, this was not what the trial was studying, but nonetheless, it was sufficient to trigger the mass consumption of selenium by men concerned about their prostates. To confirm the effect, a huge trial called SELECT was set up in the USA looking at two supplements – selenium and vitamin E. After recruiting 30,000 men, who were allocated either one or other supplement, both, or neither in a blinded fashion, the trial was stopped by the Data and Safety Monitoring Committee. By this point, the men had been followed for an average of 5 years. The Committee found that not only was there no suggestion of any benefit from either agent but, more troublingly, there was the possibility that there was a slight increase in risk of prostate cancer with selenium and, unexpectedly, the possibility of an increased risk of diabetes with vitamin E.

Even this is not necessarily the last word on the topic, however. In North America, dietary selenium levels are relatively high, hence extra may not be as useful as it would be in Europe where dietary selenium levels are lower (the difference relates to selenium levels in the soil in which vegetables are grown). In addition, selenium can be supplied as a pure chemical form or as what is known as a 'complex' linked to organic compounds more akin to the form obtained from food. Thus all we really know for sure is that the precise form of tablet used in the SELECT trial does not prevent prostate cancer in North American men. Other trials are still ongoing with both agents – for example, our own group is studying both selenium and vitamin E in men and women with early bladder cancer (also linked to lack of both in the diet) to see if supplements can prevent recurrence of the cancer.

My own opinion is that in most cases in the developed world, the levels of most vitamins and minerals will be adequately provided by most diets, particularly given the growing tendency to over-consume calories. Any effect from supplements in this setting is likely to be small, as most diets will already contain an excess over what is really needed. This is why definitive trial proof has been so difficult to obtain. As with many things in life, what starts out looking quite simple gets more complex the closer you look at it. This uncertainty, of course, fuels the market in supplements – what could be safer than taking extra 'natural' vitamins and minerals? If the men in white coats (though, of course, mostly we don't wear them any more) are not sure, why not take them just in case?

What about herbal remedies? These are, of course, attractive in the sense of being somehow more 'natural' than harsh, chemically produced pharmaceutical products. The logic is, however, intrinsically flawed – there is nothing inherently 'nice' about the natural world – watch any wildlife television show for confirmation of this. The word really has no meaning in this setting – context is everything. For example, botulism is a highly unpleasant, sometimes lethal, gut infection, but botulinum toxin is used to make people look more 'beautiful' and is certainly relatively safe as a medicinal product. The medicinal product is therefore much safer than its 'natural' source. If a herbal remedy works, it is of course because it is a drug (or more precisely, a mixture of many drugs, with varying activities and side effects).

There is also nothing magic about it being ancient (as if the length of use somehow confers an aura to it). Good examples of long-used natural remedies include witch hazel (which contains abundant salicylic acid, better known as aspirin), the opium poppy (the source of morphine and diamorphine), and foxgloves. Foxgloves are a good example of an ancient source of drugs. A brew known as 'Shropshire tea' made from foxglove leaves was used for centuries to treat the ailment known as 'dropsy' – accumulation of fluid in the lower limbs, accompanied by shortness of breath, now known to be heart failure. Then 20th-century science isolated the active ingredients – a family of chemicals named after the plant – digitalis alkaloids, of which the most commonly used is called digoxin. These drugs still form a major component of the treatment of heart failure. As far as I am aware, though, no one still uses Shropshire tea in place of digoxin.

So what about herbal cancer drugs? Well, firstly, many cancer chemotherapy drugs are indeed herbal extracts – vincristine, used to treat blood and lymphatic cancers, is derived from the periwinkle plant. The taxanes, used for many cancers including breast, prostate, and lung, are derived from the yew tree bark and leaves, and so on. Hence the study of the properties of herbs has been a major and fruitful source of some of our most potent drugs. Again, the natural source of these drugs would not make a good herbal medicine – for example, eating yew leaves is both difficult (they are very tough) and potentially fatal – the window between useful treatment effect and lethality is small.

There are examples of herbal medicines that have been tested in studies. One that I am particularly interested in is the mixture initially called PC-SPES (which stands for Prostate Cancer-*spes*, from 'hope' in Latin). This was allegedly produced from an 'ancient' Chinese herbal remedy, and marketed for 'prostate health'. Around 20 years ago, it was apparent that patients in mainline prostate cancer trials who happened also to be taking PC-SPES were deriving benefit from the herbal remedy. Despite its name, it was never tested by its makers as a cancer therapy but was licensed as a food supplement. Subsequent laboratory investigation confirmed that PC-SPES behaved like an oestrogen – technically, a phyto- (meaning plant) oestrogen. It will be recalled that oestrogens are widely used in prostate cancer therapy, and thus it is entirely plausible that PC-SPES would have anti-prostate-cancer effects. Detailed study of patients taking the mix demonstrated effects on male hormone levels and the prostate cancer marker PSA consistent with a hormonal basis for action. The clinical and chemical analyses were published in the *New England Journal of Medicine*, probably the world's premier medical journal.

This publication prompted the setting up of a trial comparing PC-SPES with a real oestrogen called stilboestrol in patients with advanced prostate cancer. The trial commenced but was stopped early due to minute levels of contamination of PC-SPES with stilboestrol. Botanic Laboratories, the manufacturers, were then shut down by the regulatory authorities in the USA, ending any possibility of completing the study. There are puzzling aspects to this story. PC-SPES had been made for years with no adverse inspections, and analysis in the original *New England Journal* article had found no contamination with stilboestrol. Furthermore, the trial, in so far as it was completed, suggested that PC-SPES was superior to stilboestrol, a result incompatible with the clinical effects being due to stilboestrol contamination, as has been suggested by some commentators.

The problem with agents such as PC-SPES is that they are only licensed as foodstuffs and hence not subject to the sorts of evaluations that a drug will have to go through. Also, the preparation is a mixture of herbal extracts, raising the question of how many components of the mix are actually required for the undoubted clinical effects seen (which included some of the known adverse effects of oestrogens such as deep vein thrombosis). The example of Shropshire tea and digoxin illustrates the potential route of development. Unravelling this would, of course, take many years and many healthcare dollars, possibly with no patent protection to allow the company to fund these costs. We will probably therefore never know what the real active ingredients are in PC-SPES. Furthermore, although the agent looked to have clinical value, it is no longer available, though a number of similar agents (called by various names, including, in a direct reference to PC-SPES, PC-HOPE) have appeared on the market and are widely used by patients. Whether these PC-SPES clones are really the same as the original, again, we will never know. With patients taking these largely unsupervised, there is no consistent body of literature on dosing, adverse effects, and so on. In addition, as these are mixtures of herbs, even if the components by weight are the same, there is no guarantee that the actual active components will be the same in consecutive batches – anyone who has a garden will know the variation seen from year to year in the plants they grow in the same bit of ground. It is hard to see any coherent way forward given the nature of herbal remedies and the current licensing environment. Companies are unlikely to queue up to carry out trials in the future of their herbal remedies given what happened to Botanic Labs with PC-SPES. Equally, the costs of turning a herbal mix into a regular drug with potentially no patent protection seem prohibitive. The pharmaceutical industry will, of course, continue to screen herbs for useful drug properties, but the subsequent development will be aimed at a single chemical entity not a herbal brew. I suspect that these agents will be forever in a shadowy hinterland between conventional medicine and alternative practitioners. This is unfortunate, as mixed in with the large numbers of ineffective therapies such as mistletoe extracts, there will undoubtedly be agents with potentially valuable activity such as PC-SPES.

In conclusion, complementary and alternative medicines form a large and economically important activity in the health economy. However, direct evidence of benefit for most such therapies is hard to find. Furthermore, in some cases, there is good evidence of *lack* of benefit. Despite this, a large proportion of cancer patients use these treatments as adjuncts to (or in some cases, in place of) their conventional therapies. Alongside these quasi-medical interventions, there is a further arena of altered diets, supplements, and herbal remedies, again largely with little or no evidence base. Understanding usage of these treatments is important as they may confound the results of trials in cancer therapy and also may interfere with outcomes from conventional therapy, either for better (rarely, probably) or for worse.

Further reading

General considerations

There are many books about cancer on the market, mostly split between books aimed at patients and their carers and books aimed at health professionals. I do not propose to list books in the first category as they are extremely numerous, needs are personal, and also vary by country of residence. I have listed books on the technical side, and again these vary hugely – the needs of a nursing student are different from the sort of reference tome required by an oncology researcher or consultant. I have split the list into reference books and more accessible paperback works.

Detailed reference books

Vincent T. DeVita, Theodore S. Lawrence, Steven A. Rosenberg, Robert A. Weinberg, and Ronald A. DePinho, *DeVita, Hellman, and Rosenberg's Cancer: Principles and Practice of Oncology*, 2 vols, 8th edn. (Philadelphia and London: Lippincott, Williams & Wilkins, 2008). This is a very substantial textbook covering all aspects of cancer from causation to treatment of specific diseases.

Edward C. Halperin, Carlos A. Perez, and Luther W. Brady, *Perez and Brady's Principles and Practice of Radiation Oncology*, 5th edn. (Philadelphia: Lippincott, Williams & Wilkins, 2008). Another comprehensive text giving in-depth coverage of the technical background to radiotherapy and the detailed clinical application by disease.

Leslie H. Sobin, Mary K. Gospodarowicz, and Christian Wittekind, *TNM Classification of Malignant Tumours: UICC International Union Against Cancer*, 7th edn. (Chichester: Wiley-Blackwell, 2010). Cancer cases are categorized using standardized systems to allow comparison of results from different studies. This reference book gives the most widely used classification system for all the recognized groups of cancers.

Bruce Alberts, Alexander Johnson, Julian Lewis, Martin Raff, Keith Roberts, and Peter Walter, *Molecular Biology of the Cell*, 5th edn. (New York: Garland Science, 2008). Probably the definitive reference book on cell biology.

Robert A. Weinberg, *The Biology of Cancer* (New York: Garland Science, 2006). Probably the definitive text on cancer biology by one of the world's leading cancer researchers.

M. P. Curado, B. Edwards, H. R. Shin, J. Ferlay, and M. Heanue, *Cancer Incidence in Five Continents*, vol. 9 (Lyon: International Agency for Research on Cancer, 2009). Detailed reference book on patterns of cancer incidence.

More accessible shorter textbooks

Terrence Priestman, *Cancer Chemotherapy in Clinical Practice* (London: Springer, 2008).

Anthony J. Neal and Peter J. Hoskin, *Clinical Oncology: Basic Principles and Practice*, 4th edn. (London: Hodder Arnold, 2009).

Margaret Knowles and Peter Selby (eds.), *Introduction to the Cellular and Molecular Biology of Cancer*, 4th edn. (Oxford: Oxford University Press, 2005).

Betty Kirkwood and Jonathan Sterne, *Essential Medical Statistics*, 2nd edn. (Chichester: Wiley-Blackwell, 2003).

Trisha Greenhalgh, *How to Read a Paper: The Basics of Evidence-Based Medicine*, 4th edn. (Chichester: Wiley-Blackwell, 2010).

Nicholas Bosanquet and Karol Sikora, *The Economics of Cancer Care* (Cambridge: Cambridge University Press, 2010).

Other reading

Ben Goldacre, *Bad Science* (London: Harper Perennial, 2009).
A superb exposé of the world of alternative medicine and quackery.

Websites

I have not included recommended books for patients and carers as these are rather a personal thing. For recently diagnosed patients, or those seeking information for relatives or other loved ones, the best initial source is probably the Internet, as information there is likely to be up to date and accurate, if sensible websites are used as sources. Factors to be considered when looking at websites should include the provider of the information. In particular, is the site selling or supporting a viewpoint or is it independent? Many large private hospitals, particularly in the United States, put up sites that include information for patients but may be biased towards treatments they themselves provide. Charities are less likely to be biased in this regard as they should have no financial interest in treatments, but may be slanted by fundraising needs. Government-backed sites may have different agendas again, perhaps with a need to downplay demand for expensive emergent therapies. It is also worth noting that treatment patterns (and hence emphasis) will vary somewhat by country; for example, surgery is the mainstay of therapy for advanced bladder cancer in most countries but accounts for only about half of the treatments in the UK. With all this in mind, it is worth consulting a few websites to compare information. Suggested initial sites:

CancerHelp UK (www.cancerhelp.org.uk/) (accessed 21 January 2011). UK-based site supported by Cancer Research UK with comprehensive information on all aspects of cancer and its treatment. The site includes a listing of all trials recruiting in the UK. The site is written in plain English for a lay audience but is multi-layered, allowing considerable depth of information. The site includes links to websites in other languages and countries.

The US National Cancer Institute (www.cancer.gov) (accessed 21 January 2011). Very comprehensive site with, of course, an American perspective. Includes a large clinical trials database for those seeking entry into a study. Also includes information in Spanish, as well as educational materials, and sections for physicians.

"牛津通识读本"已出书目

德国文学　　　　　　儿童心理学　　　　　　电影

戏剧　　　　　　　　时装　　　　　　　　　俄罗斯文学

腐败　　　　　　　　现代拉丁美洲文学　　　古典文学

医事法　　　　　　　卢梭　　　　　　　　　大数据

癌症　　　　　　　　隐私　　　　　　　　　洛克

植物　　　　　　　　电影音乐　　　　　　　幸福

法语文学　　　　　　抑郁症　　　　　　　　免疫系统

微观经济学　　　　　传染病　　　　　　　　银行学

湖泊　　　　　　　　希腊化时代　　　　　　景观设计学

拜占庭　　　　　　　知识　　　　　　　　　神圣罗马帝国

司法心理学　　　　　环境伦理学　　　　　　大流行病

发展　　　　　　　　美国革命　　　　　　　亚历山大大帝

农业　　　　　　　　元素周期表　　　　　　气候

特洛伊战争